"In this gem of a collection of stories about care at the end of life, Rabbi and Chaplain Michael Goldberg restores the spirits of his patients (and readers) as he deftly navigates from the intensive care unit to the nursing home, from a patient's home to their funeral. Across cultures and religious traditions, with steady doses of humility, wisdom, compassion, and humor, Goldberg's words are a healing balm to the often spiritually uncomfortable journey of dying."

—NASSIM ASSEFI
Internist and global women's health specialist, author of *Aria*

"With rare honesty and humility, Rabbi Goldberg welcomes the reader to accompany him into the pain-filled world of patients and families at the edge of life. He overcomes the real-world challenges of the hospital or hospice stay to bring a measure of compassion and comfort to those who suffer. Proverbs teaches that, 'The heart alone knows its bitterness.' In truth, Goldberg is that rare individual who understands the pain of another's heart and has the ability to ease that pain."

—RABBI SHELDON PENNES
Director of Spiritual Life at the Los Angeles Jewish Home

"This book is not smarmy! The stories are so gripping that you won't want to put them down. Essential reading for all who care for the dying, including their families."

—NANCEY MURPHY
Professor of Christian Philosophy
Fuller Seminary
author of *Bodies and Souls, or Spirited Bodies?*

"These remarkable stories not only reflect the experience of many dying patients, but allow readers to accompany Rabbi Goldberg in his journey of becoming a Chaplain. He reveals his own search through openly sharing his thoughts and feelings. Any Chaplain, caregiver for the dying, or simply a human being on a quest to understand what this life is all about will benefit from reading this book."

—JUDITH EIGHMY, RN, BSN, CHPN
Hospice Consultant
Pacific Healthcare Consultants

Raising Spirits

Raising Spirits

Stories of Suffering and Comfort at Death's Door

MICHAEL GOLDBERG

CASCADE *Books* · Eugene, Oregon

RAISING SPIRITS
Stories of Suffering and Comfort at Death's Door

Copyright © 2010 Michael Goldberg. All rights reserved. Except for brief quotations in critical publications or reviews, no part of this book may be reproduced in any manner without prior written permission from the publisher. Write: Permissions, Wipf and Stock Publishers, 199 W. 8th Ave., Suite 3, Eugene, OR 97401.

The Revised English Bible. Copyright © 1989 Oxford University Press and Cambridge University Press.

Cascade Books
An Imprint of Wipf and Stock Publishers
199 W. 8th Ave., Suite 3
Eugene, OR 97401

www.wipfandstock.com

ISBN 13: 978-1-55635-878-4

Cataloging-in-Publication data:

Goldberg, Michael, 1950–.

    Raising spirits : stories of suffering and comfort at death's door / Michael Goldberg.

    xii + 146 p. ; 23 cm.

    ISBN 13: 978-1-55635-878-4

    1. Death — Religious aspects. 2. Bereavement — Religious aspects. 3. Death. I. Title.

BL504 .G63 2010

Manufactured in the U.S.A.

To Stephanie,
who saved my life

Contents

Acknowledgments

WRITING THIS BOOK HAS felt at times like living with a chronic disease, and, on occasion, with a potentially fatal one at that. But thanks to the care many people gave me and this project along the way, I have managed to survive it, and I am truly grateful for their support.

First, I want to thank those "closest to the bedside," whose ongoing attentive reading made the volume better: Renee Huskey, Stephanie Kane, Sheri Katz, Nancey Murphy, Sheldon Pennes, and Richard Vance. Moreover, the work owes a debt that can never be repaid to Phyllis Gorfain for her numerous astute comments and suggestions; they made the book strong where it was weak, and where it was strong already, even stronger still.

I also wish to express my gratitude to the generous souls who encouraged me when my own spirits needed raising: Nassim Assefi, Chris Brewster, Todd Brewster, Judah Dardik, Judy Eighmy, Annie Erker, Matthew Goldberg, Nathaniel Goldberg, Edye Golden, George Greenfield, Jerome Groopman, Cathy Grossman, Kelly Hughes, Alison Jordan, Marty Kahn, Shane MacKay, Mariam Naini, Ingrid Perlongo, Helen Rolfson, Gerson Schreiber, Brian Shapiro, Archie Smith Jr., Dan Weiner, and Marc Wilson.

Finally, I must recognize one more name: God's. Without God's help, provided through all the abovementioned individuals, I could never have completed this book. Words alone cannot convey my appreciation.

1

Antawn's Voice

ASunday afternoon in the early fall and as the on-call chaplain covering a 500-bed acute care hospital in the San Francisco Bay Area, I was by myself again. Not exactly by myself, though. Walking the corridors with me was the nagging question, "What do I do if . . . ?"

Not that I hadn't already had considerable pastoral experience. I had received rabbinic ordination some twenty years earlier and had subsequently served various congregations. But hospital chaplaincy was different. The most obvious difference perhaps was that the bulk of the people whom I saw were not Jewish. Not so obvious, however, was that most of them had no idea I was. Given my last name, the failure of patients and their families to identify me as Jewish still sometimes astounds me. I am nevertheless grateful for their failures, because some of them might have concluded that since I was a Jew (something I never hid if asked), I couldn't possibly have furnished them, as non-Jews, with adequate spiritual care. But in drawing such a conclusion, they would have been just plain wrong.

For they would have been too easily equating religion with spirituality. While our various religious heritages may contribute to our spirituality, our spiritual lives as individuals may well extend beyond them. For many people—myself included—religious traditions, with their concrete doctrines and practices, are precious indeed; they help provide us our identities and orientations to the world. But in an avowedly secular culture such as ours, not everybody is "religious" in this way. Nonetheless, every human being is spiritual. By "spiritual," I don't mean something so emotionally private as to be inexpressible, or so mysteriously ethereal as to be otherworldly. Instead, I take "spirit" in a very this-worldly way, in the ordinary way that we talk about "team spirit" and "spirited horses." Spirit, in this sense, refers to anything that makes for liveliness. It's about what enlivens and animates us, what gives us a zest for living, in other words, what generates our desire to live at all.[1]

The engine sparking that passion for living differs, of course, from human being to human being. Serious illnesses and hospitals can easily dampen, if not altogether douse, a person's spirit. A patient's distressed friends and relatives acknowledge that notion every time they leave the room following a visit and whisper to one another, "She was in low spirits today." Even hospitals themselves unwittingly concede that conception of spirit by the euphemism they use to record a patient's death: Expired— literally, "the spirit has gone out."

A chaplain tries to help bring back a patient's spirit when it has been taken hostage by the pain, fear, and depression that are disease's cohorts. For me, chaplaincy offered the opportunity to learn how better to reclaim and revive spirits—and not just those of others, but of my own besides. At least for a few years, I wanted to see what providing spiritual care would be like in the focused, intense settings of hospitals and hospices. Through its stories of patients, families, friends, and staff trying to respond to the persistent knocking coming from death's door, this book recounts what I

---

1. In his book, *Christian Life and Practice: Anglican Essays* (Eugene, OR: Cascade, 2009), Owen Thomas makes a series of penetrating historical and linguistic observations about the use and abuse of the term "spirituality"—particularly in the way that it has rather recently been contrasted to "religion," much to the detriment of the latter. According to Thomas, "spirit" in English (perhaps under the influence of the empiricists) took on a narrow meaning, referring only to religion, and then, solely to religion's non-cognitive— i.e., emotional—components. But in all of the Germanic and Romance languages, "spirit" encompassed the whole range of human cultural enterprises and capacities, from politics and philosophy to science *and* religion. Hence, concludes Thomas, "The upshot of [such a] definition is that spirituality is universal and not optional. All people are spiritual. Hitler is just as spiritual as Mother Teresa. Spirituality can be good or bad, life-entrancing or life-destructive. Thus spirituality should not be used as an honorific but as a descriptive term" (cf. 19–21). I agree with Thomas's understanding of "spirituality"—and so does my use of the term throughout the book.

On that score, I couldn't disagree more with various New Age and other contemporary usages of "spirituality" that create a dichotomy not only between it and religion, but between it and rational thought. Lampooning such a notion, the satirical online journal, *The Onion*, reported the following story: "BOSTON—Father Clancy Donahue of St. Michael Church told reporters that while he believed in blindly adhering to the dogma and ceremonies of his faith, he tried not to get too bogged down by actual spirituality." *The Onion*, May 5, 2010. I am indebted to Charlie Collier for calling my attention to this article.

glimpsed of both suffering and comfort, and more than that, of repairing, restoring, and raising spirits.[2]

At first glance, a hospital's Intensive Care Unit (ICU), Critical Care Unit (CCU), and Emergency Room (ER) hardly seem the best places to undertake spiritual quests. People imagine that such pursuits require years spent in prayer and meditation in spots conducive to that sort of thing while bound for a long time to some spiritual guru or master. By contrast, ICUs, CCUs, and ERs are not venues for forging long-lasting bonds. Patients generally move in and out relatively quickly, due to discharge or death. Consequently, a hospital chaplain, like an ER physician, never knows who might suddenly come crashing through the door in need of urgent care and then, having received it, just as swiftly move on, dispatched to someplace else. More stressful still, because spiritual support is not as easily (i.e., as technologically) well-defined as "life support," a hospital chaplain never knows for certain whether he or she can provide the care required if called upon to do so at a moment's notice.

But as I walked the halls that fall Sunday and the minutes of my 24-hour on-call ticked by, I started to feel at ease: no urgent pages to the Psych(iatric) Ward, to the Neonatal Intensive Care Unit (NICU), or to the ER—just the usual requests for support, prayer, or a priest to offer Roman Catholic communion. To fill the time, I began "self-rounding" in the CCU and ICU, areas specifically assigned me for daily coverage during the week. "Self-rounding" means taking the initiative to visit patients who had at least not indicated their refusal to see a chaplain. In a society in which so many people have had distasteful experiences with religion, fleeing its "organized" forms in droves, chaplains have to take seriously that a patient's "No" means "No!" Both hospital policy and genuine religious humility demand no less. Still, in an age of ever more cost-conscious hospital administrators who might jump at the chance to write off pastoral care as a dispensable "frill," chaplains need continually to justify their

2. The book's stories are not "merely" stories: they are, every one, drawn from real cases. In every case, however, I have changed the names of the persons involved—patients, families, and caregivers, both professional and lay—to protect their confidentiality; indeed, in a few circumstances, I have added some elements further to conceal, and thus to protect, their actual identities. Much of the key dialogue in the book is verbatim, and in those instances when it is not true word-for-word, it nevertheless truthfully reflects what was said.

existence by keeping their patient census up. Thus, "trolling for business" is a necessary part of a chaplain's job, and a unit's charge nurse usually provides the best leads.

I made my way to the ICU and swiped my hospital ID card through the electronic lock on its doors, pushed them open, and walked over to the charge nurse's station. Charge nurses strike me as master sergeants, commonly sharing the same no-nonsense air of authority.

Properly obeisant, I asked in hushed tones, "Do you think there's anyone who could use a visit?"

Sergeant Nurse surveyed her domain, flicked her hand in a direction behind and to the left of me, and brusquely replied, "That patient over there had a tough visit this morning with Dr. Booth."

The charge nurse was referring to the intensivist, the physician with primary responsibility for the ICU, and Dr. Booth, I knew, was a doctor genuinely devoted to his patients. The nurse went on to explain that Dr. Booth had wanted this particular patient, who had AIDS, to take his prescribed anti-viral drugs; otherwise, he would have to go on a ventilator. Then Sergeant Nurse gave me my assignment. "So far, this man won't do the obvious, simple thing and just take the drugs. You're a chaplain. Maybe you can get him to take them—or at least find out why he won't." Having assigned me my mission, my NCO handed me my marching orders: the patient's chart.

Eager though I was to embark on my assignment, I knew that reading the chart could impede as well as aid me. Due to its highly clinical, technical focus, a medical chart can transform the person described as well as the person reading that description. It can metamorphose the former into a sheer disease and the latter into a mere medic. Even so, a chart's "H&P"—the section recounting the patient's "History and Physical"—may offer a chaplain at least an introduction to a stranger's story. Whether it provides an accurate introduction is another story altogether.

The patient, reported the chart, was a forty-six year old African-American male who had been diagnosed with AIDS fours year earlier after having tested HIV-positive eight years prior to that. This year, the H&P continued, he had developed an esophageal ulcer that had become increasingly more severe. Finally, according to the chart, when, two days earlier, the patient had spiked a fever of 103 degrees and had suffered acute dehydration as a result, his primary physician had had him admitted to the hospital.

After I finished reading the chart at the nurse's station, I turned around to look for the man's room. "Room" is a misnomer in the ICU and CCU. Most patients' "rooms" in those units are not really rooms at all. Instead, they are more like berths on a train, little bed areas separated from a main hallway by curtains. No curtain, however, enveloped my patient's bed. Instead, glass encased his space, and a sign taped on it warned: "Tuberculosis Risk! Put On Mask Before Entering!" I reached for a nearby box of surgical masks.

Sergeant Nurse barked, "Not those! The ones with the double straps!"

Having been duly instructed and unduly mortified (two results only charge nurses can achieve with remarkable effectiveness and regularity), I obediently picked up the proper mask. Then I noticed I also had picked up two escorts, anxiety and dread. "Just how contagious is he?" I wondered. "Do I have the mask on tight enough?"

As I entered the cubicle, I saw my patient for the first time. I noticed he was wearing a mask of his own for oxygen and lay in bed almost completely prone. A young white woman sat at his bedside. Turning to the patient, I said, "Hello, I'm Michael. I'm a chaplain on this unit. I come around every day to visit folks."

I tended to introduce myself in such broad terms to leave wide openings for patients to respond however they wished. While I might assist them on their spiritual journey, the course had to be theirs, not mine. Therein lay for me chaplaincy's attraction as well as challenge. Patients could lead me to a spiritual landscape that, but for them, I myself might never envision, much less enter.

For this particular patient and me, however, our first step was more of a stumble than a start due to the masks we were each wearing. Through his oxygen mask, the man grunted, "What? What did you say?"

I realized that my surgical mask had muffled my voice and hidden my face as much as his oxygen mask had stifled his words and partially concealed him. Besides that, the damn surgical mask had made my glasses fog and was making it hard for me to breathe normally. And then it struck me: the man lying before me wasn't the only one in that room with impaired, diminished capacities. But what then of my other mask, my professional persona as "Hospital Chaplain"? How could I possibly function in that role when I couldn't use any of my usual props—my voice, face, and eyes—to help me pull off my performance?

Nevertheless, the curtain had gone up, and the show had to go on. I tried to start the conversation again. This time, I put considerably more effort into making myself heard distinctly. "My name is Michael. I'm a chaplain here. Is there any spiritual care or support I can give you?"

The man, too, appeared to put more energy into making his voice heard. "I just want God to get me through this."

"What do you mean by 'this'?" I asked.

Did he mean facing the choice, as the charge nurse had supposed, of either taking the anti-viral drugs or going on the ventilator? Or did he mean enduring, or perhaps, more basically, even surviving his current hospital stay? Or did he mean something else entirely? Although his words were clear enough, their meaning seemed anything but transparent.

"I don't understand" I pressed, not giving the man a chance to respond as my anxiousness and mission drove me forward. "Could you just say a little more about what you mean?"

But he merely answered, "For God to just be with me."

I took his response as an evasion, as a type of "spiritual cliché" disguising some deeper unresolved issue. I turned to the young woman sitting by his bed, thinking she might be of help. I had not really acknowledged her thus far, and I thought that if nothing else, trying to converse with somebody else in that glassed-off space might at least make me feel a little better.

"I'm sorry. My name's Michael. What's yours?"

"Suzanne."

"How do you know each other?"

"We're members of the same church, Lighthouse Witness in San Francisco. He's the best singer in our choir!"

The church, with its charismatic pastor, was known not only as among the most racially mixed and socially active in the city, but also as its most musically gifted and energetic. For the first time, the man before me became more than a patient: "The best singer in our choir." Now that singer lay in front of me, barely able even to speak, his voice weakened by disease, choked by an oxygen mask, and soon possibly silenced altogether by a ventilator. Although I already knew his name from the chart, I felt the need to have him speak it; to hear him say it was a way of prying open a passageway to his identity as he himself understood it. Our names, after all, provide the most concrete moorings on which to build the bridges of our individual identities to those around us.

"What do your friends call you?" I asked.

"Antawn," he replied.

Looking for a way to learn more about him, I inquired, "Antawn, if you could wish for one thing right now, what would it be?"

"To sing again."

How many times have I heard seriously ill patients wish for something other than what many would guess the clear-cut choice, namely, just to get well? Maybe the gravely ill know that is too much to ask, and that therefore a request like Antawn's is much more "realistic." The very sick are frequently, in fact, much more realistic than their families, their friends, and, at times, even their physicians. I decided that Antawn's desire to sing once more, despite his current condition, may have appeared to him more achievable than restored health, let alone full recovery.

Trying to be supportive, I interjected, "Well, you know today *is* Sunday. Maybe we could have a little service with some singing right now."

Too late, I caught myself. "Oh my God!" I thought. "What have I done? What if he asks *me* to sing some hymn?"

A Christian hymn *per se* did not pose some theological "issue" for me. I just didn't know any Christian hymns, at least not well enough to lead one. My professional mask, it seemed, was being lowered more all the time. *I* was supposed to be the spiritual caregiver; my official hospital badge as much as said so: "Pastoral Care Department." Despite that, I was stumped.

With controlled desperation, I turned to Suzanne. Summoning up all the smarminess only a trained religious type can muster, I "invited" her to start us off, "Perhaps you could lead us in a hymn, Suzanne."

She wasn't much help, either. "I'm blanking."

"Don't panic, don't panic, don't panic," I told myself.

Trying to act encouraging while simultaneously attempting to make sure the task didn't fall back on me, I asked her, "Well, what did the choir sing in church this morning?"

Suzanne looked over at Antawn and said, "Oh, they sang the one for Imogene." Imogene apparently was another severely ill member of the congregation. "You remember this one?" Suzanne asked as she began singing the verses of a hymn I had heard before, "Leaning on the Everlasting Arms." Unexpectedly, I found myself somehow moved.

When Suzanne stopped, I asked Antawn if there were other hymns he would like to hear. He mentioned another, this time one I didn't know at all. Suzanne began to sing again, and for the first time, I became conscious that she, too, was wearing a surgical mask. What actually made me aware of that was not any dampening of her voice beneath the mask, but of her dampened eyes behind it.

Antawn may have noticed her eyes, too, because in the middle of her singing, he blurted out, as much as he could "blurt" anything from under his own mask, "Oh, that's enough!"

Smiling, Suzanne acknowledged Antawn's good-natured teasing. "It sounds like you need to get back and lead the choir again real soon."

In that moment, Suzanne and Antawn had managed to raise each other's spirits—and mine, too. Often, that's all spiritual caregiving is: raising spirits. Raising someone's spirits does not, of course, make that person "all better." It does not magically furnish any healing that is once-and-for-all. Instead, raising a person's spirits provides a momentary spark of life, an evanescent sense of being alive at a time when such a sense may be needed most—and yet in the long run, it is not nearly all that's needed.

In a fleeting instant, the rare, precious moment shared by Antawn, Suzanne, and me was gone. Besides, Antawn's voice had grown increasingly fainter. Before I got up to leave, I asked Antawn if he needed anything else.

"Just for God to get me through this."

There it was again. That straightforward but still maddeningly enigmatic answer. What did he mean by "this"? Now, however, was not the time to ask. I would have to return another time to learn more.

I asked Antawn if it would be all right if I said a prayer before I left. Exhausted, he could only nod. He, Suzanne, and I reached for one another's hands. I tried to gather up the strands of the words spoken and sung in the twenty minutes we had spent together.

"God," I began, "please let your friend, Antawn, feel your everlasting arms around him. Let him not only feel you, but hear you in his heart to give him the guidance and clarity he may need for his life. Give him the voice to sing again, but most of all, let him hear your voice through what Jesus says in the gospel when he speaks his good news, 'I will be with you always.'" Suzanne said, "Amen." Antawn squeezed my hand.

Emerging from the cubicle, I virtually ripped off my mask, happy to breathe normally again and to feel my body relax. In the next second, though, both my breathing and body tightened up once more as I realized to my dismay that I had failed in my mission assignment. Bad enough that I hadn't gotten Antawn to change his mind about taking the new drugs, worse yet that I had no more insight now than prior to my visit about his reason for not taking them, but worst of all, I had never even raised those subjects with him in the first place! My chart note reflected how far short of my objective I had fallen:

> Per RN referral, I visited pt. and friend in attempt to help pt. get clearer about his future treatment.... Offered support and prayer. ... Per availability, will visit pt. again to follow his progress in gaining clarity about the life choices currently open to him.

Finishing my note, I resolved to return to Antawn's cubicle a couple days later in my medical gumshoe role and see if I could turn up some clues.

But when I came back, Antawn was asleep. Nevertheless, my sleuthing was not entirely fruitless, because during that visit, I met somebody who cracked the case for me. My informant's name was Moira. Like Suzanne, she knew Antawn from church. In her twenties, green-eyed, relatively tall, she had long, light-brown hair. An office worker in San Francisco, she told me she had been Antawn's long-time friend and, over the past two and a half years, his caregiver too. I learned that even now, she drove across the bay to visit him each day during her lunch hour, though given the distance and the traffic between her office in San Francisco and our hospital in the East Bay, I was sure the time it took her must have well exceeded an hour, by any measure. To me and anyone else willing to take the time to listen, Moira cogently explained Antawn's resistance to taking the antiviral drugs recently recommended for him.

Some months previously, Antawn had had a bad reaction to an AIDS cocktail prescribed by his primary physician, whom he saw but once a month. When he tried to tell her about the drugs' side-effects during their subsequent monthly meeting, the doctor had responded, he thought, with virtually no empathy at all. As a result, a fresh mix of drugs with potentially adverse reactions coupled with several weeks' wait to see his apparently unsympathetic physician did not appeal to him—nor would it, I think, to any reasonable person with Antawn's first-hand, twelve-year experience of his illness.

Imagine my surprise, then, when at the start of our visit together the very next day, Antawn began by saying, "If I got to have the drugs, I got to have them."

I was so thrilled by the news that I could hardly wait for the visit to end so that I could report back to the medical staff: "Mission Accomplished!" I charted Antawn's decision verbatim, orally reported it to Dr. Booth, the intensivist, and even left a note at the charge nurse's desk for Antawn's primary physician to page me (something, by the way, she never did).

Not much later, however, a blush of embarrassment replaced my flush of victory when I cooled down and recognized that although I may have performed superbly as a member of the "interdisciplinary medical team," I had failed miserably as a chaplain. For one thing, I had never stopped to ask Antawn exactly *why* he had changed his mind. Moreover, I had ignored his initial cryptic requests for God to be with him and to get him through "this" every bit as much as his primary physician had earlier ignored his complaints about the side-effects of her prescriptions. Finally, while the hospital staff afforded Antawn all kinds of physical caregivers—three daily shifts of them in fact—I was the only staff person it specifically offered him for spiritual care, and I had been shamefully negligent in that capacity.

As much out of a sense of guilt as anything else, I decided to keep visiting Antawn. I wanted somehow to make up for my "spiritual mal-practice." But a sense of curiosity also drove me. What concretely was it that Antawn wanted from God? How would he actually know if God were really "with" him? And whatever "this" was, what would it mean for God to get him "through" it?

Unfortunately, hospital realities stymied my good intentions. The next time I went to visit Antawn in the ICU, he was no longer there. He had improved enough to be transferred to a less acute unit I didn't routinely cover. It was another chaplain's coverage area, and turf and boundary issues are sometimes sadly as much a part of a hospital's pastoral services as they are any other piece of its larger bureaucracy.

Soon, however, Antawn was back with me in the CCU due to another hospital reality: a patient's improvement or decline is seldom linear. In the space of a few short days, his condition had again taken a downturn and with it, any chance of our carrying on a conversation together. His voice was now choked both by a ventilator and heavily sedating drugs. During my first two visits, he had spoken with me only briefly. Over the next fifteen times I went to see him in the succeeding three or four weeks, he barely spoke half a dozen sentences and none of them consecutively.

Therefore, much of what I learned about Antawn, not only about his life itself, but also about his beliefs about his life, necessarily came from others, chief among them Moira. She was devoted to him. She continued to visit him virtually every day, and, through the course of several talks with her, I learned that her judgments about Antawn and his feelings were more reliable than anybody else's. Who could explain the connection between Antawn and Moira? It wasn't racial. He was black; she was white. Nor was it sexual. He was gay; she was straight. In retrospect, the best word to characterize their bond might be "sacred."

I am hesitant to use that word in a culture that has so little sense of things holy that it seems almost hell-bent on profaning them through trivialization, from Madonna's dabbling in *kabbalah* to bumper stickers' sloganeering "WWJD?" In such a context, Moira's sitting by Antawn's bed day after day displayed something sacrosanct, even numinous. In keeping her faithful daily vigil at Antawn's bedside, Moira seemed to vividly embody God's assent to Antawn's prayer "to just be there with me."

Had I continued to view Antawn's situation through the prism of the powerful medical culture so prevalent throughout the hospital, it would have been easy for me to construe Moira's continuing presence at his bed each day as "clinical denial" of what was happening. But that daily bedside image of her with Antawn instead made me see something else instead: my own "spiritual denial." That denial had led me to dismiss, out of hand, the plain meaning of what Antawn had asked of God the first time we met. Why had it been so hard for me to take Antawn's words at their face value, that is, in terms of their spiritual values? Ironically, what may have blinded me to what Antawn was saying was the set of interpretive lenses I had picked up during my seminary training.

Back then, my classmates and I had to take a course in pastoral counseling taught by one of New York's premier psychiatrists. One day in class, he asked us, "Suppose you're visiting a hospital patient who says to you, 'I know I'm here because God is punishing me!' What do you say in response?"

Before giving anybody in the class a chance to respond, he answered his own question: "You must say right away, 'No, that isn't true!'"

The psychiatrist's canned rejoinder did not spring from some theological conviction about God's role in illness and healing. Rather, it reflected his belief that psychotherapy, and psychotherapy alone, could alleviate a patient's anguish. Thus, sitting in that classroom, we little rabbis-in-training were led to see ourselves not as people, who in calling on the ill, were performing the traditional *mitzvah* of *bikkur cholim*, the religious obligation of visiting the sick, but as para-therapists ever alert to interpreting professed spiritual responses as symptoms of deeper psychological issues. Only years later would I figure out the right initial response to a patient perceiving sickness as God's punishment: "What makes you say that?"

No wonder, then, that Antawn's first replies to me failed to reach me. Given the mission Sergeant Nurse had assigned me, my old self-image as a would-be psychologist had re-emerged and virtually re-absorbed my more recent self-understanding as a chaplain. Moira's sacred presence at Antawn's bedside reminded me that my chapel was not some shrink's office, but a patient's room. In Antawn's room, in the presence of him and Moira together, I recognized that I was on holy ground. Like all revelations, mine was in part self-revelatory, for it showed me not only the answer to Antawn's prayer, but also the implications of my professed vocation if I were to care properly for him and others like him.

Caring properly for Antawn meant understanding his own sense of his life's meaning. Moira was the source of that revelation, too. She told me that when Antawn had learned twelve years earlier that he was HIV-positive, he made a vow to God that he would dedicate his life to becoming a servant of God by serving others so long as God let him live. That vow was what filled him up. In that sense, it *inspired* him with virtually the breath of life of itself. It gave him the spirit to struggle on through long periods of suffering. That vow to God made twelve long years before was the source of Antawn's feistiness, his spiritedness, in short, his spirituality.

Antawn's room displayed the way his vow had shaped his life, for the small space enclosing him always bulged with cards, pictures, prayers, balloons—and visitors. And what a diverse group of people squeezed around his bed! Black and white, young and old, gay and straight, all coming to visit a man who barely spoke, frequently just lying there largely "out of it" due to the breathing tube down his throat and the heavily-sedating medications given him to tolerate the tube.

Neither pity, nor mawkish sentiment impelled Antawn's visitors to come see him. Rather, a sense of respect drew them to a man who had persistently shown care for many of them in the past, often when nobody else would, not even they themselves. One young man, for instance, told me, "A few year ago, Antawn grabbed me by my lapels, shook me, and screamed at me to start getting right about my life, starting with getting off dope. Since then, he's been like a father and a brother to me, depending on which one I needed right then. Antawn always just seems to have the right sense about that sort of thing."

Other visitors also testified to Antawn's impact on their lives. A quartet he had helped organize years before came to serenade him in his room, much to the delight of many staff members—and to the exasperation of Sergeant Nurse. One day, the leader of the church choir showed up and said its members wanted to add their voices in support of Antawn. But gathering all its members in his small space was clearly out of the question. The choir therefore threw a benefit in Antawn's honor at a civic auditorium. Several hundred people attended, paying fifteen dollars and up for tickets, the proceeds of which went to Antawn's ever-rising medical bills. The first time I had met him, Antawn had expressed his wish "to sing again." Now, his breathing tube, his drugs, and his worsening condition conspired to make the fulfillment of that wish less and less likely. But his voice had not been totally silenced, either. Through the devotion reflected in the singing of the quartet and choir and in the support of friends and family, the distinctive moral and spiritual timbre of Antawn's voice echoed mightily.

I myself was unable to attend Antawn's benefit concert because it fell on a Sunday when I had to take call yet again. Monday, I was eager to hear all about the benefit, but I first got some distressing news from Dr. Booth. When we passed Antawn's bed on rounds, he motioned slightly in Antawn's direction and whispered, "He's treading water in a bad place." I knew that, of course, but hearing Dr. Booth say it made me more conscious of it than I wanted to be. A couple of days later on my own rounds, I came upon Moira in the corridor outside the CCU. "I was at a patient care conference this morning with Antawn's mother, sisters, and doctors," she told me. "Antawn said that if his heart stops beating, he doesn't want to be brought back."

I was stunned by Moira's words. But what stunned me even more was my being stunned at all. I certainly did not disagree with Antawn's decision to be designated as a Do Not Resuscitate (DNR) patient. I thought it was the right decision. And yet, a flood of questions filled my head. How could a man so strong just give up? What about his vow? If he was supposed to dedicate himself to God's service so long as God let him live, then why not give the hospital's technology a chance to revive him so he could continue fulfilling his part of the deal? Then I caught myself. Such questions, I realized, were merely my weak attempts to cloak my own sorrow about losing Antawn. The first time I saw Antawn, my professional mask had proved of little benefit. The more I continued to see him, the less value it seemed to have to me.

"Moira," I asked, "did anyone at the care conference discuss home hospice so Antawn might at least die in familiar circumstances?"

"No," she answered, "but I'll ask his primary doc about it tomorrow."

I wasn't surprised that no one had discussed hospice, nor was I optimistic that anyone would recommend it as a next step in Antawn's care. If many physicians view death as a checkmate in the contest to save a patient from a disease's ever-encroaching onslaught, then hospice signifies their forfeiting the match altogether. Thus, when I saw Moira next day and she told me that Antawn's doctor had advised against taking him home, I was hardly shocked. Nevertheless, on rounds soon afterwards, I made it my business to talk to Dr. Booth myself about the matter. Without mentioning my prior conversations with Moira, I asked him about the feasibility of sending Antawn home to die.

Standing outside Antawn's cubicle, the intensivist looked over at his patient, then back at me, and said, "He's on the edge. I doubt he could even survive the ride across the bay. Let's see, though, if we can move his bed outside to the fourth-floor patio so he can get in the sunshine at least one more time in his life."

I felt a little better—until Dr. Booth quickly added, "But you know, his preferences will soon become less and less important to him."

Dr. Booth was right. Three days later, Moira told me, "Antawn really doesn't care where he dies now. Moving him in any way, even turning him in bed, causes him so much pain."

Another patient care conference ensued. A prior commitment to meet with another patient and her family prevented me from attending it, but later, I read the chart note reporting its outcome: "Pt. desires to continue current aggressive supportive measures."

I suppose some at the conference, perhaps chief among them his primary physician, found Antawn's decision puzzling, even infuriatingly perplexing. From what Moira had told me, that doctor, in particular, had been the one at the earlier care conference who had had the most trouble telling Antawn that further treatment would be futile. But then, she had also been the one whose own futility in getting him to follow her drug regimen had originally led certain staff to designate him "non-compliant." For her and those like her, that label may well have still seemed quite fitting in terms of Antawn's decision-making. How could a patient want, on the one hand, to be DNR while on the other elect to continue aggressive life-support?

Only Antawn's spiritual commitments could resolve the apparent inconsistency. Antawn had made a promise to serve God if God would keep him alive. So long as God kept him alive, Antawn intended to keep his part of the covenant between them by serving God in any way he could—including as a dying man in a bed in the CCU. To Antawn, clinging to life in such circumstances provided evidence, *physical evidence*, of his commitment to keep faith with God by rejecting anything that might hasten his death. *But* when death finally did arrive through *God's decision*, Antawn viewed resuscitation as every bit as faithless as having his life ended by the premature removal of life support. In the last analysis, only Antawn's spiritual framework, and not, for instance, some psychosocial one, could explain his apparently contradictory decisions about his treatment—and explain, in the process, the meaning to him of *both* his life and death.

I had prayed many times for Antawn over the past several weeks, sometimes when the two of us were alone in his room, sometimes when visitors were there with us, at times when he was alert, at others when he was asleep. I had also prayed for him at home by myself. But for a few days following this last patient care conference, I did not know what kind of prayer to speak to God. To let Antawn die quickly? To sustain him? And if so, how?

At a loss, I once more turned to Moira for guidance. She took out a slip of paper on which she had scrawled a prayer the night before, sitting at Antawn's bedside during one particularly frightful three-hour period when he did virtually nothing except cough and gasp for air. Moira handed me the prayer scratched out in that time of utter helplessness for both of them:

"God, allow him to stay or allow him to go. Allow him whatever journey it is that You have been preparing for him ... and for us."

"And for us." None of us knew what course God might lay out for Antawn. All I knew was where Antawn's journey had taken me so far. It had forced me down a hard road, making me see how easily I could lose my way as a chaplain. Regaining my bearings had required my first getting a true heading from Antawn, whose spiritual compass had repeatedly shown itself to be more reliable than mine.

That Sunday, I had another on-call rotation. This time, it was anything but routine: pages to the Psych ward, to the NICU, and to the ER to cover a death in the middle of the night. When Monday finally came, I felt like a patient relieved to be going home to recuperate. Returning to work Tuesday, I felt refreshed as I went into the CCU to make the morning rounds.

Antawn's bed was empty. He had died the night before.

I felt a double loss. One was Antawn's, of course. But I grieved as well the loss of those who had come to see him all those weeks, people I would never likely see again. I felt myself bereft of a community of comfort in whose midst I might find some consolation.

And then Moira called. She always appeared, it seemed, when I needed her most. When I needed insight into Antawn's perspective on his living and dying, she had been there; when I needed guidance in prayer, she had been there once more; now, when I needed solace, there she was again. Not that she had ever appeared in any dramatically "religious" way, spouting Scripture or the like. Instead, she had a way of simply *being there* for Antawn, for me, and for who knows how many others like us. And who can say? Such simple presence may be the way God is largely among us, too.

Calling from her San Francisco office, Moira said, "We've planned a memorial service at the church this coming Sunday. We'd like you to be part of it."

"Thanks very much," I answered. "I can't tell you how much it means to me to be invited. Let me see if I can get off and come."

My response was less than truthful. I was touched as well as honored to be invited to the service. But I didn't really need to see if I could get off that Sunday because I had not been scheduled to work then. I just had reservations about going to the service.

Early on in chaplaincy, either someone else's experience or your own teaches you not to grow attached to patients. Patients, after all, are not your family, nor do you generally spend enough time with them to form lasting friendships. Visiting critically ill patients and desperate families in intense circumstances can easily lead you (and them) to confuse such intensity with intimacy. And grieving deeply the loss of every patient finally results in being unable to serve any.

And yet, if no patient's death ever truly pains you, the result will ironically be the same, namely, the inability to truly serve any patient, because then there will be no patients, only "cases." Mere "cases" *per se* cannot be patients, much less human beings. In that sense, no chaplain—and, I would add, no doctor, nurse, or social worker—can genuinely serve a "case." To those nonetheless insisting that patients *must* be viewed as "cases" to receive appropriate treatment in medical facilities, my response is simple: Fine, there are always "special cases." For me, Antawn was a special case and more. For Antawn made me reflect on *myself* as "the case" to be studied, diagnosed, and in some way healed. Going to Antawn's memorial service was part of that healing.

But although I had decided to attend the service, I still had some misgivings about leading part of it. My hesitancy had little to do with being a Jew participating in a Christian service; it had a lot to do with being a Jew who had little idea what to offer in a church service that would surely be emotionally exuberant. What could I say to catch the spirit of the occasion and thus do my part to raise the spirits of Antawn's family, friends, and the congregation itself? A friend of mine says that the spiritual life is largely unexplored territory.[3] Small wonder, then, that I felt myself on unfamiliar terrain without a map. Like it or not, however, I was already well underway in this current expedition, and so when the pastor's office called a day or two later to invite me again to lead some part of the service, I felt I had no choice but to accept.

When I arrived at the church that Sunday for Antawn's memorial, the pastor hardly helped me feel more at ease. He greeted me curtly, even coldly. Perhaps, I tried to reassure myself, his mind was just racing ahead to the countless details attendant on the actual business of managing such a large service. I know my own mind has strayed on similar occasions, sadly leaving behind those mourners to whom I should have been the most attentive at the time. Or maybe, I reasoned, the pastor has cultivated the stern detachment of a biblical patriarch in order to maintain order among his unruly flock consisting of large numbers of homeless people, recovering addicts, and runaway teens. Or conceivably, it suddenly

---

3. The friend is Prof. Theophus Smith of Emory University, and for this characterization of the spiritual life as well as for the above-used phrase, "spiritual malpractice," I am indebted to him.

dawned on me, Antawn simply had not meant as much to the pastor as he had to me and the others I had met. For the pastor as for me, just as for every other human being, individual lives and deaths affect us, John Donne notwithstanding, in very different ways.

At last the service started, and how else could it have possibly begun but with music from the choir? Given the breathtaking quality of its singing, I could only imagine how magnificently Antawn himself must have sung to have been deemed, as Suzanne had said in his room a month before, "the best singer in the choir." After the choir completed its opening selection and took its seat, the pastor got up and welcomed everyone. He then introduced the associate pastor, who after speaking a few minutes, in turn introduced me.

As I moved toward the pulpit, I wished I could speak with the same fervor bordering on abandon that appears at times to fill black churches. But I could only speak with a Jewish voice, and even among the most fervent Chassidic Jews, our liturgical voice is characterized by order rather than abandon. Indeed, the Hebrew word for prayerbook, *siddur*, and for the weekly Torah reading, *sedrah*, both stem from a root that means "order." It is through such order that, for better or worse, Jews' souls sing. Had I tried to make my soul resonate then in a voice other than a Jewish one, I would have struck a false note. And so I began with the words of Job 1:21 with which the order of every Jewish funeral service traditionally begins:

"The Lord has given, the Lord has taken away: Blessed be the Name of the Lord."

And then I followed the assignment I had been given by the pastor prior to the service. Unlike the misguided—and misleading—assignment Sergeant Nurse had originally given me, the charge the pastor bestowed on me was the right one for a chaplain, and more important, the right one for me. For the pastor had given me nothing so broad as a eulogy nor so narrow as a psalm. Instead, he had simply asked me to offer "some words of comfort." I realized that I could not offer comfort to the mourners in the church unless I first acknowledged myself as one of them, as one in need of comfort, too. Now in the face of Antawn's death, my professional mask had been stripped away entirely. That meant speaking not as "officiant," nor as professional consoler, but as another mourner talking broken heart to broken heart:

"I have been asked to give a prayer of comfort. It begins as a prayer of thanksgiving for the comfort you, Antawn's family, friends, and community, have given me and the other hospital staff who cared for Antawn—and I mean *cared* for Antawn—by inviting us to be with all of you here now so that we, too, can begin to be consoled and healed. Thank you Antawn's mother and all the family, thank you Moira and all the caregivers, and, of course, thank you pastors and all the members of this church, for reaching out to us.

"And thank you, God and Antawn.

"God, thank you for the gift of Antawn, who gave so much for his part to the rest of us by the way he embraced his life—and confronted his death. He showed, he physically and spiritually displayed, he *witnessed* to your faithfulness to him and his own faithfulness to you in kind. As many of you already know, over twelve years ago, Antawn made a promise to serve God with his life so long as God sustained his life. So long as God kept his end of that covenant between them, Antawn intended to keep his part as well, to serve God in any way he could, even as a dying man, often in agony in the Critical Care Unit. To keep his word, Antawn refused to accept any measures that might hasten his death and thus relieve his pain. It makes me think of Mark 15:23 describing Jesus on the cross: "Then they gave [him] wine mingled with myrrh to drink [to dull the pain], but he would not take it." Antawn's witness, like Jesus', would let God, and God alone, decide how and when he was to die.

"The first time I saw Antawn in the hospital, he asked that God just be there with him to get him through this. And God ultimately did just that—by enabling Antawn to keep his word despite his suffering. Someone once told me that Antawn always seemed to have the right sense about what somebody needed most at the moment. Maybe Antawn sensed that the example of his life and death are what we'd be needing most at this moment. In the midst of our suffering, may we come to know that God is and will be there to get *us* through this, too. Amen."

Grasping the significance of Antawn's mask during my first encounter with him had unmasked me by making me aware that he wasn't the only impaired one in that little glass cubicle. So, too, this last contact with him brought home to me, as I took my seat, something else too often overlooked. Sometimes, prayers for healing are not merely for the sick, but for us, the pray-ers also.

"And for us."

2

Tenagne's Breath

I LIKED THE QUIET of the Chaplains' Office first thing in the morning.
Some days, I had no other sacred space to prepare myself for the hospital's pandemonium.

By chance, I had arrived for work a little earlier than the others in
our office, a Quonset hut set apart from the hospital proper and situated
on not the safest street in the uneven neighborhood roundabout us. I
delighted in my sanctuary's solitude and stillness as I walked through its
narrow corridor to the small kitchen in the back. I put on a fresh pot of
coffee, and then, waiting for it to brew, returned up front to the office's
computer where I logged on to the list of patients admitted overnight
who had requested a chaplain's visit. I scanned the screen for those I
had responsibility to cover, specifically, those patients sent to the ICU
or CCU as well as any Jewish patients assigned to the hospital's other
units. Undistracted, I copied down my patients' names, together with the
numbers of their rooms and beds, until the aroma of the by-now brewed
coffee wafting through the office lured me back to the kitchenette. There,
I reached up into a cabinet for the ceramic mug I kept on hand with the
tranquil image of *Christina's World* imprinted on it, filled it to its lip,
poured in two packets of artificial sweetener, stirred their white crystals
into the steaming pitch-black potion, and sat down to savor both the coffee and the moment.

It was not to be.

The five-note, off-key electronic scale of my pager shattered the serenity. Its small window flashed "5233," the ICU's extension. The coffee
splashed onto the desk as one hand smacked down the mug while the
other plucked up a phone. The ICU line answered after a single ring.

"This is Michael Goldberg at the Chaplains' Office," I said. "I'm responding to your page."

"We need you up here *stat!*" squawked an unfamiliar female voice.

"I'm on my way," I said, knowing the only response that mattered to an ICU page was the one I had just given. Explanations, details, the whole backdrop for any drama that might unfold, would have to await my arrival on the unit's floor.

As I started to lock the office's front door, I saw one of the other chaplains coming toward me on her way to work. I rapidly told her where I was going and then bounded up the block-and-a-half of sidewalk between our office and the hospital, straight through its automatic doors—only to be thwarted by its elevators, their mechanisms seemingly designed for leisurely voyagers on ocean-going liners rather than for restive travelers on frenetic rides up-and-down. Even when I finally caught an elevator for my trip to the fourth floor and the ICU, it seemed determined to slow my progress toward my destination, laying anchor at each level where its doors would sluggishly let on and off its passengers of visitors and staff.

When the doors opened on the fourth floor and my turn came at last, I dashed out and darted toward the ICU. With each advancing step I took, shrieking from farther down the hallway reverberated nearer me, its source apparently the waiting room located just outside the ICU itself. Usually a domain of silence ruled by the kind of dread that suppressed speech of any sort, the anteroom was today anything *but* that. As I passed it to swipe my ID badge through the electronic sensors on the ICU's locked double doors, I glimpsed nearly a dozen women with skin so dark it looked blue-back, their number complemented by half again as many men, the entire contingent standing, sitting, even squatting to scrunch themselves into every inch of the tiny room's cramped quarters.

I went inside the ICU and, after asking around, found the nurse who had paged me.

"Hello," I said, "I'm Michael Goldberg from the Chaplains' Office. How can I help?"

Without giving me her name in kind or so much as looking up, the nurse started reading notes from off her clipboard. "Twenty-year-old woman, recent Ethiopian immigrant, came in last night to give birth. In delivery, she threw an embolism. She's brain dead," the nurse reported. Then, tilting her head toward a glass cubicle to her right, she added, "She's hooked up to a ventilator over there. The husband's going to have to sign a consent to take her off it—we need the bed." And *now* came the reason for the nurse's paging me. "To top it all off," she said with rising exasperation, "their relatives out in the waiting room are making such a racket, they're upsetting the families of the other patients we've got in here. See what you can do!"

Virtually no amount of clinical training or experience could have prepared anyone, whether an unsympathetic nurse or an empathetic chaplain, for the scene that greeted me as I entered the ICU waiting room outside: explosive ululating, ferocious breast-beating, even garment-tearing, all accompanying a language whose very phonemes struck my ears as utterly alien. But amid the commotion, a slender young man stood stationary with head bowed and hands folded against his chest, his sole movement the fluttering of his lips. Although I hated to intrude and interrupt his prayer, he appeared my lone point of entry into territory so completely foreign.

"Excuse me," I said gently, "I'm Michael, one of the hospital's chaplains. Is there anyone here I can help?"

The young man lifted up his head; I could see he had been crying. "Thank you," he said softly. "My name is Alemu. You can pray for my wife, Tenagne." Then he slowly pointed toward the ICU, "She's in there. They say she's dead. But God can do miracles, just like Jesus did with Lazarus." He took a breath, as though to stifle a sob upwelling from deep inside. "So, please, Chaplain Michael, pray for my Tenagne."

My theology concerning miracles and resurrection did not matter—what counted was comforting Alemu, and *that* meant learning more not only about him but also about his life together with Tenagne. "Of course I'll pray," I replied. "However, I'm afraid they haven't told me much about your wife or what happened to her."

Never quite raising his eyes to meet mine, the soft-spoken man waited again before he answered. "Please forgive my English. Amharic is what I grew up speaking at home in Ethiopia, just like everyone else you see around me. Like them, Tenagne and I came here not long ago to escape the problems of our country—many, many cruel things were being done to people there. Getting out was not easy. It took bribes, and it meant leaving the rest of our family behind.

"Then we found out we were going to have a child—a boy!—and we were so happy, Chaplain Michael, because here in America, he could have a better life. When Tenagne's time came yesterday evening, I brought her to the hospital. She is young and strong. They told us everything would be fine with our son's birth—but then they said something had gone wrong, that Tenagne had died, and that our son's life was in danger. That was at two last night; now it's after eight this morning. While I've been staying here, our community has gathered to be with us." Alemu concluded his story as he had begun it. "Please, Chaplain Michael, pray for my Tenagne." As before, I said, "Of course."

But why had Alemu not asked me to pray additionally for his son, whose life might still hang in jeopardy? Maybe he regarded the child not merely as some stranger, but as the very one responsible for the death of his beloved wife. For now, though, questions about the inner workings of Alemu's mind had to come second to those concerning his community's public practices and shared beliefs.

"Alemu," I asked, "do you belong to a church? Is there a minister or priest I can call to come and pray with us? Is there a friend or somebody in your community I should contact?"

"We are Ethiopian Orthodox; someone has called His Eminence to come, and, thank you, but the proper person in our community has also already been notified."

"His Eminence"? "The proper person in the community"? Who were these people, and how might they be of help to Alemu—and to me? I wanted to ask Alemu more, but he had turned away in tears, engulfed not only by his own weeping but in an instant by the heightened wailing of his community, whose members, as though one vast wave of lamentation, billowed up and over him as he descended, coming to rest cross-legged on the floor.

Aware that I lacked even the minimal knowledge to give me the footing necessary to scale the mountain of issues confronting me, I realized I had no choice but to return to the base camp of our office to make provision for what might lie ahead. So I made the trek from the ICU back through the fourth-floor corridor to the elevators, enduring another long wait for one, followed by an even longer downward ride, before legging it back up the stretch of sidewalk leading to the Chaplains' Office. By now, it had been transformed from my own private chapel into the whole hospital's "Pastoral Care Department," its staff transfigured from a single cleric into a full complement of "Spiritual Care Providers," all of them awhirl readying themselves for their daily rounds while, at the front desk, a secretary was hard-at-it handling the incessantly-ringing phones.

Each chaplain had a cubbyhole that overhung a five-yard tabletop we used in common. I scurried past the other chaplains' cubbies to my own nook and pulled down from it the object of my journey: a spiral-ringed paperback entitled *Culture & Nursing Care: A Pocket Guide*.[1] The foot-high, inch-thick booklet had always served me well as a primer on multi-ethnic patient care. Running the gamut from Brazilians to Hmong to Russians as well as to many other nationalities and groups, its chapters sketched each one's perspective on subjects ranging from "Food Practices" to "Illness Beliefs" to "Death Rituals," the topic so significant to my present purpose.

I turned to the chapter headed "Ethiopians and Eritreans."[2] It both reflected and illuminated what I had previously witnessed in the ICU waiting room. Contrary to the ICU nurse's sentiments about the Ethiopians' graphic show of grief, such a display in Alemu's community was to be encouraged rather than extinguished. Indeed, from what I read, some cultural gaffe, exceptionally grievous in every sense given the circumstances, had likely set it off. Among Ethiopians, according to the handbook, news of a loved one's death ought never to be communicated to a family member except through a close friend. But who had probably brought Alemu the grim tidings about Tenagne? Almost certainly a harried physician, culturally-uninformed at best, culturally-uninterested at worst, and in either case, impatient to have Alemu disconnect Tenagne from the respirator.

Better equipped now to help than when I first arrived, I again traversed the various distances, both horizontal and vertical, that separated our office from the waiting room outside the ICU. The expressions of misery that met me there had lost none of their explosiveness, as though almost powerful enough to burst the walls themselves. I took a deep breath and waded into the crowd, hoping somehow to find Alemu amidst the turmoil. As if from nowhere, a woman, slightly older than Alemu but every bit as lean-limbed, interposed herself between me and the others in the room. "I am Mahelet," she said, "and I will tell Alemu whatever it is you have to say." Her voice had the same softness as Alemu's, but it con-

1. Juliene G. Lipson, Suzanne L. Dibble, Pamela A. Minarik, eds., *Culture & Nursing Care: A Pocket Guide* (San Francisco: University of California Press, 1996). At the outset, culture is defined as "a system of symbols that is shared, learned, and passed on through generations of a social group. [It] mediates between human beings and chaos . . . and guides people's interactions with each other. It is a process rather than a static entity and it changes over time" (1).

2. Eritreans are not a separate cultural but political group within Ethiopia. For this point as well as several others in this paragraph, see ibid., 101–14.

tained an assertiveness his did not. Apparently, I now stood face-to-face with "the proper person in the community" designated by Alemu (and the handbook) as the correct conduit for communication.

"My name is Michael," I responded, "and I'm one of the hospital's chaplains. Thank you for coming so quickly. I have to admit I don't know much about your community or its ways."

"They called me," replied Mahelet, "because I, among them, have lived here the longest. I came six years ago, and I own an Ethiopian restaurant in the neighborhood. Besides," she quipped with a faint smile, "my English is better than theirs." Growing serious again, she inquired, "Tell me what has happened. I arrived here only a little while ago, and I know few of the details of what has taken place."

I repeated to Mahelet everything I knew concerning Tenagne's condition, explaining that during delivery, a clot had formed cutting off the blood flow to her brain, irreversibly ending its activity, and thus medically, at least, her life. I tried to make my explanation as simple and straightforward as possible, not because I thought Mahelet unintelligent, but because I could not imagine the prowess required to convey, in *any* language, the full meaning of my words to someone as overwhelmed by shock and desolation as Alemu. I searched Mahelet's face for comprehension. "This much," she said, "the hospital has already told Alemu. Still, though, he wants to pray to God to help Tenagne."

"I know," I replied. "When Alemu first spoke with me, he mentioned that 'His Eminence' had been called. Who might that be?"

"That's the Bishop," Mahelet told me. "He's a very important figure in our community, which also makes him a very busy one. It may take him quite some time to get here, but I doubt Alemu will do anything until he does."

I looked up at the clock in the waiting room, and it was already after ten. By the time I looked back down, Mahelet had disappeared into the sea of mourners, gone perhaps to find Alemu and relay what I had said. Without her, I felt myself at sea, adrift both linguistically and culturally among all the Ethiopians. But as soon as I spun around to search her out, she bobbed up again in front of me, Alemu firmly in tow. Her resurfacing brought in its wake something else quite unexpected: near-silence in the waiting room.

"I told them to lower their voices," Mahelet said. "In our country, their crying might be normal, but here, it distresses others."

"Chaplain Michael," Alemu interjected, "have you prayed for my Tenagne yet?"

"No," I answered, "I wasn't really sure about your church's custom, and I thought we might want to wait for His Eminence to come and offer the prayer himself."

"None of us knows when His Eminence will come," Alemu countered, "but my Tenagne needs a prayer right now. So will *you* go and pray for her?"

"Why don't we *both* go?" I suggested. I had a pair of reasons for making my proposal: I wanted to get a closer look at the faith Alemu kept in prayer's life-sustaining power—*and* I needed him to take another look at the contraption keeping Tenagne artificially alive.

Leaving Mahelet in the waiting room, Alemu silently followed me into the ICU. Tenagne lay in the first glassed-off enclosure to our right. As I beheld her for the first time in her glass case, she reminded me, despite the ventilator tube protruding from her lips, of a Sleeping Beauty cast under some witch's spell. Next to me, Alemu wept all but imperceptibly. "Let's go inside," I said, "and sit down with Tenagne."

As we entered the cubicle, I took its two chairs and placed them flanking Tenagne's bed. Alemu and I sat down across from one another, each of us holding one of her hands in ours, he transfixed by her face, I riveted by the rhythmic groaning of the respirator and her chest's too-regular rise and fall. "Alemu," I said after several minutes had gone by, "because I don't know how your church prays, why don't you start out the prayer, and then I'll finish it?"

"Thank you, Chaplain Michael, I would like that," he replied, genuinely grateful.

He bowed his head, clasped Tenagne's hand, if possible, still more tightly than before, and, eyes shut hard, brought it to his forehead. "Holy Miryam, Mother of God, please help my Tenagne. We both believe that your son, Jesus, gave life to Lazarus, just like God gave life to him—even when everybody around them said that they were dead.

"Now, everybody here says Tenagne is dead. Please, Mother Miryam, have Jesus and God prove them wrong. Please have them, we beg you, give life to my Tenagne."

A few tears rolled down Alemu's cheeks as he opened his eyes and looked at me. Although I would follow his prayer's lead, mine would split off onto another path that would bring us to a different end point.

"Lord of all flesh," I began, "we recall Scripture's story of the Shunnamite woman's child, whom everyone took for dead. But through your prophet Elisha, you miraculously resuscitated him and brought him back to life.[3] Resuscitate Alemu's dear Tenagne, Lord, and restore life's breath to her."

I took a breath before continuing. "And yet, God, we recall something Scripture also tells us—that our lives here on earth are like a breath, our days as fleeting as a shadow.[4] At this moment, we know that all too well. So should it not be your will, Lord, to resuscitate Tenagne here on earth with us, we ask that you resurrect her nonetheless in heaven, alongside you and Jesus and all the saints."

In a voice that barely registered a whisper, Alemu said, "Amen."

A quarter hour must have passed before Alemu spoke again. "Thank you, Chaplain Michael," he said. "Let us wait and see what God does for my Tenagne."

I thought that in the interim, the two of us should go and see what God was doing elsewhere. "Alemu," I ventured, "have you thanked God for the breath of life he's given to your son?"

"No, Chaplain Michael," Alemu answered, staring sheepishly at his shoes like some Sunday-school miscreant. "I haven't said any prayers for him as yet."

For *him*? In light of the tragedy surrounding Tenagne's delivery, I wondered whether Alemu had any feelings whatsoever for his newborn child.

"Alemu," I offered, "why don't the two of us go down to the hospital nursery, look in on your son, and give thanks to God for him?"

"But what if something happens here with Tenagne?" Alemu objected.

"I'll tell people where we're going and to page me if anything develops," I replied.

I informed the charge nurse where we were headed and to have me paged if Tenagne's condition changed; I next located Mahelet in the waiting room and, more in an effort to reassure Alemu, told her the exact same thing. Reluctantly, Alemu followed me down the corridor, repeatedly glancing backwards toward the ICU. Bypassing the elevators, I led him

---

3. See 2 Kgs 4:8–35.

4. Cf. Ps 144:4.

down two flights of stairs to the nursery, intent not so much on saving time as on sparing him any more anxiety or guilt about leaving Tenagne's side.

The landscape of the nursery could not have been more unlike that of the ICU or its waiting room, for here, delight rather than disquiet reigned. I peered through the nursery's oblong window at the babies, three rows deep, each with his or her own blue or pink little cap and booties. Despite myself, I couldn't help but contrast the infants in their Plexiglas bassinettes with Tenagne in her glass alcove: their lives, however fragile, had gotten underway while hers had reached its end.

"Alemu," I asked, "which child is yours?"

He pointed to a baby boy, squealing and squirming as vigorously as any other tyke around him. I was relieved to see the child apparently stabilized and thriving.

"What have Tenagne and you named him?" I inquired.

Alemu averted his eyes, whether in shame or not I couldn't tell. "We haven't yet given him a name. Since last night, there's been no time for that."

"Look down at the band around your wrist," I prompted him. "It has your last name on it. Remember? You and Tenagne each got one right after the baby was born. He, too, is wearing one that identifies him as yours. We can show the nurse your wristband, and then she'll bring your son to us so we can offer a prayer thanking God for him and asking God's blessing on him now and in the future."

"No!" recoiled Alemu. "We can say the prayer from here!" At that instant, I realized that for Alemu, holding his son meant letting go his wife. In his mind, embracing the infant, its very being so plainly full of life, entailed accepting Tenagne's death, her body little more than a balloon of artificially-pumped air. To Alemu in his present state, the baby represented not Heaven's blessing but its curse.

"As you wish, Alemu," I said as I laid my hand upon his shoulder. "If you like, we can pray for your son like we did for Tenagne: you start it off, and I'll conclude it."

"No, Chaplain Michael, you say it all."

When we had prayed earlier for Tenagne, Alemu had bowed his head and shut his eyes together tight. Now, he stared straight ahead, his gaze overshooting his baby altogether, landing instead on the nursery's back wall. I pondered what I ought to pray. For the baby's sake, I wanted to summon words that would acknowledge and affirm him.

"Lord God," I eventually began, "we haven't yet given this little boy a name. But to you his identity is already known: he *is* your gift to us. We thank you for your gift.

"May this gift of yours, this little boy, continue to receive your blessing as he grows up, and may he receive the blessing of others, also. Let him give blessing to their lives, too. We therefore pray, God, that throughout his life, he be recognized as a blessing-bearer, among your most precious gifts of all."

His body quivering, Alemu murmured, "Amen." After that, he turned around and walked out of the nursery back to the main hallway. When I rejoined him, he simply asked me, as if in a daze, "Chaplain Michael, how do we get back to Tenagne?"

I led him to the stairwell, but from that point on, I followed *his* lead: he sprinted as much as climbed the stairs up to the fourth floor, where he ran toward the ICU and Tenagne's bedside. As I raced past the waiting room, I heard no keening—Mahelet presumably had matters well in hand. Meanwhile, up ahead, the ICU's locked doors had stopped Alemu in his tracks. Reaching him, I swiped my badge and gained us access. But when Alemu took another look at Tenagne lying in her bed, tubes and all, he began bawling as uncontrollably as any babe in the nursery two floors below. He wheeled around and bolted out of the ICU; within seconds, even before I could exit the ICU after him, I heard renewed wailing from the waiting room. Stepping hesitantly inside it, I saw no sign of Alemu anywhere. As I anxiously looked around for him, Mahelet, as she had done previously, popped up in front of me without warning.

"Mahelet," I stammered, more than a little startled, "where is Alemu?"

"Somewhere over there," she answered, motioning with her arm in the direction of a pulsating mass of women huddled over, I assumed, an inconsolable Alemu. "Nothing more is to be done," she said, her voice a monotone, "until His Eminence arrives."

"But when will that be?" I pressed. "Have you received any word since we last spoke?"

"As I told you before," she answered, "His Eminence is a very busy man."

I had no reason to doubt Mahelet nor therefore any grounds to believe I could do much more at this juncture to help Alemu or, for that matter, the medical staff, either.

"You know your community and its customs far better than I do, Mahelet," I reiterated. "I believe you when you say that nothing will happen until the Bishop comes. But meantime, I have other patients and families I need to see. Please tell Alemu to have me paged when the Bishop gets here."

"As you wish," she said deferentially, though still with no detectable emotion in her voice as though she alone among her community had come to understand the full import of all that had transpired.

Close to noon by now, I finally started on my daily rounds through the ICU, the CCU, and the various sub-acute units in the rest of the hospital where I met with the Jewish patients whose names I had jotted down earlier that morning in the office, a time that now felt like ages, rather than mere hours, ago. All the while, I kept sneaking glances at my belt to make sure I had not missed a message from my pager, which I had switched to its "vibrate" mode to minimize its disrupting a conversation between some patient and myself.

As I departed one room on my way to the next, I felt an unmistakable series of tingling sensations on my hip. I let out a slight sigh of relief, believing the bishop had finally arrived at the ICU. But when I looked down at the pager's window, I saw it displaying the extension of the Chaplains' Office instead of the ICU's. I found a phone free at the nearest nurses' station and called in.

"This is Michael. Just got your page. What's up?" I asked tersely of our secretary at the other end.

"There's a Jewish family in the ER," she answered, maintaining her equanimity. "Their seventy-five-year-old grandfather has had a heart attack. They asked if we had a rabbi to come sit with them."

"Tell them I'll be right over," I said hanging up as the tension mounted in me. Despite my efforts to reign them in, my thoughts were galloping headlong toward the Emergency Room: "How long will it take to save the old man's life—or for him to die? . . . What if I'm down in the ER trying to comfort his family when Alemu's bishop arrives in the ICU, and they page me to go up there? . . . How can I be in two places at once?!"

This time, I didn't begrudge the elevator's delaying me as it laboriously made its way down to the first floor. It gave me the chance to collect myself before entering the ER's tightly-structured tumult. I got the attention of the charge nurse and inquired which family had requested me. She gestured toward a middle-aged woman, a man about her age beside her to her left, and a teenage girl adjacent on her right. All of them, unlike the Ethiopians four floors up, sat silent in their apprehensiveness.

"Anything on the patient's condition?" I asked the nurse.

"Nothing yet," she replied.

I went over to the family, introduced myself, and took a seat with them. The patient—the woman's father—had a history of heart problems; widowed years before, he lived, despite his daughter's protests, by himself in a senior apartment complex. That morning, his maid had hardly begun her weekly cleaning when he collapsed. She called 911, and the paramedics were sent, who, for their part, rushed him to the Emergency Room. I asked the family the old man's Hebrew name, and then I repeated it as I recited aloud the traditional Jewish prayer for the healing of the sick. Afterwards, I translated the prayer's Hebrew into English. From experience, I knew that for many Jews, regardless of belief, comfort resided less in the Hebrew's actual meaning than in the language's sheer sounds. In that respect, the Jews down in the ER and the Ethiopians up by the ICU resembled one another, after all: the bare vocables of the familiar consoled both of them alike.

Forty-five minutes later, an Emergency Room physician emerged from the treatment area to report that the old man's heart rate had been returned to normal and that, purely as a safety measure, he would be transferred shortly up to the ICU for further observation. The family expressed its gratitude to the physician—to which, inwardly, I added mine. The family thanked me as well, and before we parted, I told them I also covered the ICU and that, should they need me, they would likely find me there later that afternoon.

Leaving the ER, I checked my pager—no messages from the ICU or from anywhere else in the hospital. My watch, though, showed the time well past one, and I had not eaten since 6:00 AM. If I didn't grab a bite at this point, who knew when I might?

The hospital's emergency room occupied the same floor as its cafeteria, its trauma center thus conveniently located to treat the aftereffects of the convenience foods its canteen dispensed: outsized-packs of pork rinds, all manner of Hostess Products—Twinkies, Ding Dongs, and Hi Hos (not to mention cupcakes!)—and jumbo Coca-Colas. I actually once saw a wife present such fare to her morbidly-obese young husband only hours after the ER had narrowly revived him from a cardiac arrest. At the time, I wondered whether his spouse held a large insurance policy on his life—or whether some perverse hospital architect had designed a fiendish floor plan to make sure all the beds stayed filled.

Sidestepping the cafeteria's medley of artery-plugging delectables, I crossed over to its salad bar, got a tray, a plate, and silverware, pitched some greens and other vegetables together, paid for them, and spotted an open table to eat my lunch. I was picking through it piece by piece, relishing each mouthful, when—Dammit!—the pager started vibrating. I looked down and saw it blinking the ICU's extension. The bishop (I hoped) had arrived at last.

I dropped the fork back on my near-full salad plate, hoisted up the tray beneath it, and hurriedly took everything over to the conveyer belt for transport to the kitchen for clean-up and disposal. Without even considering calling back the ICU or having an elevator haul me up there, I climbed up all four flights of stairs, my anticipation (and breathlessness) growing with every step. As I approached the waiting room outside the ICU, I heard no sound at all. Perhaps Tenagne had died, everyone had gone home, and I had only been paged to comfort Alemu—and to ask for his consent to harvest Tenagne's organs, a mission that, whatever its benefits to individual patients or overall rewards to "science," I nevertheless abhorred, feeling it as ghoulish as any grave robber's.[5]

But no: I looked inside the waiting room and found it still filled with Ethiopians. Hushed, they encircled Alemu, and yet, the epicenter of the stillness was someone else, an older, thickset figure—"His Eminence." He looked every inch the patriarch with his flowing salt-and-pepper beard and full ecclesial regalia: black, red-trimmed cloak draped from his shoulders to the floor, matching black, red-embroidered mitre perched atop his head, gold-colored shepherd's crook enfolded in his hand. Positioned down the hall nearer the ICU, I noted another Ethiopian new to me, stand-

---

5. Apparently, I am not alone in that feeling. Indeed, if, as physicians claim, they are "scientists" who can always learn something from each and every autopsy, then why, one wonders, do they give consent for autopsying their own bodies or those of their family members *in percentages far lower than the general population*? What knowledge—or misgivings—do they possess different from the rest of us? See Dr. Richard P. Vance, "An Unintentional Irony: The Autopsy in Modern Medicine and Society." Online: http://www.researchgate.net/publication/20849525_An_unintentional_irony_the_autopsy_in_modern_medicine_and_society.

ing ramrod-straight as if stationed at attention, his hands locked behind his back. He wore a dark suit and tie over a white, ill-fitting shirt, its closed collar bunched unevenly about his neck.

Once more, Mahelet precipitously resurfaced. "I will tell His Eminence that you are here so that you can take him and Alemu to see Tenagne. When he has finished what he has come to do, his driver," she said, nodding toward the man in the dark suit, "will take him to his next appointment."

With that, she disappeared back into the throng, only moments later to bring the bishop out, along with Alemu close behind. As a sign of respect to the bishop—and the community whom he served—I briefly bowed my head before him. Besides, who knew if he spoke English or, for that matter, what knowledge he had of Tenagne's true condition? The bishop momentarily smiled at me, but otherwise made no reply. Meanwhile, Mahelet had vanished once again. Nothing, therefore, remained for me to do except to swipe us through the ICU's electronic doors and lead the bishop with Alemu to Tenagne's cubicle. To give them their privacy, I stayed outside it.

Through the glass, though, I could follow the prayer-in-pantomime enacted over Tenagne's bed—Alemu knuckling his hands hard into his chest, the bishop mouthing some supplication, no doubt sacrosanct and ancient. Then, the bishop's lips stopped moving, and Alemu seized Tenagne's bedrail, his body wracked by anguished spasms. Although I would have wrapped an arm around Alemu to try and soothe him, the bishop wagged a finger in his face, issuing, for all I knew, the Amharic equivalent of "Cut it out!" because Alemu immediately stopped shaking. The bishop, his duties evidently thus performed, gathered the furls of his cloak together and set forth from the cubicle and the ICU, leaving Alemu clutching Tenagne's bedrail.

I vacillated about going in to join Alemu. Maybe he needed some minutes by himself; maybe he needed some support. In the end, I simply couldn't bear to stand by any longer and watch him suffer all alone.

When I walked in, Alemu looked up, his gaze hollow from weariness and worry. "Chaplain Michael," he said piteously, "we just need to give God more time to restore my Tenagne to me."

I didn't say a word but just grasped his hand. The man indeed needed a miracle—but not the kind he had in mind. Instead, he required the heaven-sent capacity to concede that his beloved Tenagne no longer lay before him, but only her lifeless counterfeit.

For a while, we stood side-by-side there staring down, the room's silence unbroken save by the respirator's relentless droning in chorus with the unremitting pinging of the monitors around us. Then suddenly came another sound, a nonstop rapping on the glass behind us. I looked over my shoulder and saw the charge nurse insistently waving me toward her. I looked back at Alemu to excuse myself, but his eyes had never left Tenagne.

As soon as I set foot outside the alcove, the nurse planted herself opposite me, scarcely a handbreadth from my nose, and as though she were a cop grilling some suspect withholding crucial information, demanded, "So, did you get his consent to take her off the vent?"

"No," I shook my head.

"Well, I'm taking a lot of heat from the docs about it. They want the bed and the equipment back. OK, then, I'll let *them* talk to the husband and explain what's what."

"Fine," I said unenthusiastically, "but if they're going to have any chance of success, they'll need to speak to him through a go-between from his community named Mahelet."

Annoyed, the nurse replied, "And I'll let *you* explain that to the doctors when they get her. I'm going to send a page out to them now."

And so she did.

Within minutes, two practically identical physicians appeared at the ICU's nursing station: white-coated white men, well over six feet tall and, by my guess, pushing sixty, too. I sensed they shared something else as well—the stress of having been called to help resolve an issue that might well defy all the medical expertise and skill they possessed.

"What's taking so long getting the family's consent?" the first physician asked me briskly, not due perhaps to any general lack of caring or of kindness, but because like many of the hospital staff, myself included, he had nearly reached wit's end trying to slog through a crisis-laden day.

"The husband is a new immigrant from Ethiopia," I said, "and in his culture, such matters are broached through a third party, some established, respected member of the community. I have that person in the ICU waiting room right now, and I can bring her in for you to speak with. She'll tell the husband what you've said and then bring back word to you. Even then, I should warn you, the husband might not agree. He's a deeply religious man who believes that with enough prayer and time, God will reverse his wife's condition."

"Look," said the second physician, "I don't know any anything about divine interventions, only about medical ones. The poor fellow needs to face the fact his wife is *dead*. Period. End of story. Is that him in there?" Before I could say another word, off they went into Tenagne's room. Stunned, I mutely tagged behind. When the three of us entered the cubicle, Alemu appeared to take no notice.

"Ahem," coughed the first doctor, "my colleague and I are physicians here in the ICU." As though he had thus given Alemu introduction and courtesy enough, he continued, "We know this is difficult for you, but you need to accept the fact that your wife is gone. She only looks like she's alive because the ventilator is mechanically pumping air into her lungs. But the embolism she threw last night killed her; she's brain dead. There's nothing we—or anyone—can do to bring her back. We'll have the forms sent in to have her taken off life-support. After you sign them, why don't you go down to the nursery and visit what we understand is that newborn son of yours?"

Throughout the monologue, Alemu never once looked up. At its conclusion, he replied, resolute as ever, "Thank you, Doctor, but I believe in God and in his miracles."

The two physicians, their medical capabilities unable to remedy the situation, turned their stares on me, the chaplain, their message unmistakable in meaning: "*You* handle this!" Then, as one, they wheeled around, trooped out, and disappeared from view.

I knew at that moment what I wanted to say to Alemu, and I knew I had to say it *with* Mahelet but not *through* her. I went out to the waiting room, peeked in, and relieved to find her still present, stretched out my arm to signal her over toward me.

"I need you," I told her, "to go inside with me to Alemu and Tenagne. Have you ever been in an ICU before?"

Her stoicism and self-confidence, formerly so self-evident, faded before my eyes. As though transmogrified through some dark art, her bearing abruptly mirrored Alemu's—eyes downcast, shoulders stooped, a voice so distant it seemed to come from someone else's body. "No," Mahelet said, "I've never been in one of those places."

"Don't worry," I replied, "I'll be right there with you."

I led her inside the ICU. Recalling that Tenagne's cubicle already had two chairs, I carried in another from out on the unit floor, and set it by the bed so that Alemu, Mahelet, and I might sit together for the words that must be said. But I might as well have been invisible, for Alemu never so much as glanced up at me while Mahelet remained on the glass's other side, brought up short, if not totally unnerved, by the tableau composed of her compatriots and contemporaries within—a man poised motionless above a virtually dead-still woman lying with a tube twisted down her throat. I put my hand out to Mahelet, and after a few seconds' faltering, she stepped forward and took a seat in the chair I placed beside her. Next, I lightly touched Alemu's shoulder and, pulling up a second chair, indicated my desire for him to take a seat as well. I sat myself down in the third, remaining chair between the two of theirs.

"Mahelet," I asked as delicately as I could, "Alemu mentioned when I first met him that he and Tenagne came here to escape the cruel things being done to people in Ethiopia. What kind of things?"

"The government," she answered in a voice I had to strain to hear, "rounded people up for no good reason. Those they didn't kill on the spot, they imprisoned and tortured until they died."

I leaned in close enough to Alemu's face to make sure that he couldn't possibly divert his eyes from mine. "Alemu," I said, "keeping Tenagne in here hooked up to these machines is like imprisoning and torturing her— it only prolongs her dying."

I realized how hard those words might have been for him to hear; even so, I had others that might prove harder still. "Alemu," I went on, "you've told me how you believe in God and in his miracles. And I'm sure you do. But none of these machines is God: if *they* could have produced any miracles, they would have done so long ago."

Alemu slowly raised his head, opened his mouth, and exhaled no mere sigh, but something more powerful, like an uprush of air from the bellows of a heart breaking deep within. Afterwards, he simply said, "Bring me the papers. I will sign them."

And then, as she had throughout the day, Mahelet materialized at precisely the right moment, in exactly the right place, kneeling by Alemu's side. She stayed with him while I went to retrieve the proper paperwork and staff to have Tenagne taken off the vent. When the nurse handed the document to Alemu for his signature, he took it, read it through deliberatively, and then, pressing firmly on the clipboard to which it was attached, firmly wrote his name. He watched attentively as the technicians disconnected the various devices from Tenagne's body. When they finished, he turned away and said, as much to himself as anyone, "She is gone." Resignation and recognition had at long last converged. Alemu walked out of the cubicle, Mahelet not far behind.

Bringing up the rear, I hurriedly pushed my way through the ICU's twin doors toward the waiting room, more than half expecting to find the Ethiopians' rites of mourning re-ignited as Alemu shared the news of Tenagne's death. To my surprise, though, it had emptied of its occupants, whom I saw ahead of me, noiselessly tailing Alemu down the hallway leading to the elevator bank. I felt a momentary urge to overtake them—maybe they were headed to the nursery!—but then I thought better of it, lest I overstep.

Tenagne had died quickly, perhaps free of any suffering. But Alemu's torment extended well past her death—all the way to Ethiopia and back.

3

Mr. Liu's Neck and Sally's Knees

AS A GRANDCHILD OF the Enlightenment, as a child of modernity, and as an adult trained in academic philosophy, I entered chaplaincy with a host of virtual certainties about reality: events had reasons grounded in physical causality, medicine rested on science, and the world made sense because of its roots in rationality. But two cases profoundly challenged those convictions.

I was making my usual rounds in the CCU one morning when a nurse pulled me aside and said in a low voice, "You better go visit Mr. Liu. He's just received some bad news about his cancer."

Obviously, being with a patient, being with anyone, just after they've gotten bad news, is not easy. For many, if not most, of us, the natural impulse is to avoid the person or to try to say something that will make things better, words of some sort supposedly bringing comfort and solace. But shock may serve as a shield against traumatic tidings, and words may not penetrate its protective barrier. Frequently, in fact, having another human being present at such a moment is itself not a comfort but a burden. Grief for many people is the only tolerable companionship then, despite its having come uninvited. To be honest, I, too, would just as soon be elsewhere at such times. And yet, there are people who do not desire solitude at that time but company, and a chaplain's own desires take second place to theirs.

So I knocked on the entrance to Mr. Liu's cubicle and stuck in my head to introduce myself and ask if I might enter. But when I saw him, I literally came face-to-face with the last thing I expected: he was smiling. Maybe, I thought to myself, his doctor hasn't yet broken the news to him, and I sure wasn't going to be the one to do it. Or maybe his doctor *had* told him, but had bungled it so badly, Mr. Liu had not really understood the terrifying information given him. Unfortunately, there is plenty of evidence to show that physicians, for all their training, are not necessarily specialists when it comes to imparting news like that.[1] But then, I wonder if anybody is—or can be.

Grinning broadly, he invited me to take a seat, "Come in, Chaplain! I'm glad to see you."

I began with my standard question, one as open-ended as possible to see how Mr. Liu might respond and thus how and where I might follow his lead. "So what's going on today?"

"I've just received wonderful news," Mr. Liu beamed.

Although I didn't know the nature of Mr. Liu's "wonderful news," I did know I felt a huge sense of relief. At the same time, though, I also felt more than a little irritated when I thought back to what I had wrongly been told only a bit earlier about Mr. Liu's supposed diagnosis. Despite the hospital's incessant talk about its "interdisciplinary team approach to patient care" and its "cross-functional communication," it not infrequently had difficulty even getting the patient's condition passed down the line correctly. Notwithstanding modern medicine's daily reliance on high-tech equipment, we found ourselves, when it came to communication, routinely playing a form of the childhood game, "Telephone," where the original message winds up distorted beyond all recognition.

Trying to hide my exasperation as best I could, I asked, "So, Mr. Liu, tell me, what's your good news?"

"They thought I might have cancer in my spine, but there's no trace of it at all!"

"That sure is good news!" I answered affirmingly. "But what made everybody think you might have cancer in the first place?"

Mr. Liu hesitated, as though he had qualms about responding to my question. I feared I might have overreached.

Then he propped himself up on his pillows, pushed himself slightly toward me and started speaking in a soft, almost inaudible voice. "The only way I can answer what you asked is by telling you a story that might sound strange. I know you must be busy. Do you have time to listen?"

"I certainly do!" I responded without a moment's hesitation. I believe that no medical chart, no bits of abstract data, not even when given by the patient herself or himself, can tell as much about that human being as that person's own story, especially as she or he relates it firsthand. Naturally, it

---

1. Cf., e.g., Dr. Jerome Groopman, "Dying Words: What Doctors Are Never Taught to Say," *The New Yorker*, October 28, 2002, 62–71.

might be skewed, but it's always a good place to start. In fact, I think it's the only place to start.

"I have all the time you need to tell me your story, Mr. Liu, and I honestly feel very lucky that you're willing to have me hear it."

His body, which had looked so tense moments before, relaxed almost immediately as he eased himself back down on his pillows.

"I am Chinese," he began. "Among us, honoring parents is very important, especially for a son.

"Many years ago, as a much younger man, I came here to America, but I left my parents behind in Taiwan. I offered to bring them with me, but they said they wanted to stay there. So we each made our choices.

"I would go back to Taiwan once a year to visit my parents, and though we were always glad to see one another, I could also see how much they missed me, and I could never rid myself of the guilt for having left them.

"As the years passed, my parents grew older, and the older they became, the more frail they became. Of course, I went back to Taiwan more frequently to see them and to look after them as best I could. I sent them more money from here, and called their doctors, their friends, and my other relatives over there to help look after them in my place.

"Eventually, though, my parents died—actually within a fairly short time of one another, in fact; I made the trip back to Taiwan for each one's funeral.

"Still, I kept feeling guilty. I kept thinking that, as a Chinese son, I had not done enough to take care of my parents, to be with them when they needed me. My feelings of guilt lasted a long time. I even went to a therapist for counseling to help me cope with my guilt. But it persisted nonetheless. Finally, I decided the only thing I could do was to return to Taiwan to visit my parents' graves and to ask my parents for their forgiveness.

"My parents are buried in a beautiful setting. It is really quite different from the kind of cemetery you find here in the States. Their graves are nestled in a park on a hillside with a path leading up to them. At one point, the path intersects a brook and to get across, you have to walk on some stones made smooth by the water streaming over them.

"I entered the cemetery and followed the path toward my parents' graves. After making my way carefully across the wet stones in the middle of the brook, I climbed slowly up the hill and eventually arrived at my parents' resting places. I was not aware how much time I spent there, because I could only feel my shame for not having been with them more, particularly near the end of their lives, and for my sense of having failed to show them the respect owed them by their son. At last, while staring down at their graves, I asked my parents out loud for their forgiveness.

"After that, I turned and started back down the hill. I came to the brook and cautiously stepped out onto the smooth, wet stones. I crossed three or four of them. Then suddenly I slipped on the next one, fell backwards, and hit the base of my neck hard on a rock behind me.

"After lying there dazed for several minutes, I tried to get up, but I could not do it right away. The cold water had numbed my hands, and in addition, the slippery stones gave me nothing firm to hold on to. When I did finally manage to stand up, I knew immediately something was wrong. Pain shot all the way down my spine. It hurt so bad I could barely walk.

"I had a fourteen-hour flight to catch back to the States that night, and because of the tremendous pain I was in, I knew the trip might be unbearable. I did not know a doctor in Taiwan, and, even if I had, I doubted I could be seen on such short notice before my flight departed. So I stopped at a drug store on my way to the airport and bought some over-the-counter painkiller and a neck brace. Not surprisingly, they did not help much, and at times during the flight, the pain was excruciating. As soon as the plane landed and arrived at the gate, I pulled out my cell phone and called my doctor here to see if he could call in a prescription for some more effective painkillers.

"He said he would not prescribe anything for me without examining me beforehand. First, he ordered an X-ray, then a CAT scan, and finally an MRI. I must tell you, Chaplain, I was becoming very frightened. I began to think maybe I had injured myself so seriously that in the end, the doctor would bring back some kind of horrible report telling me that before very long, I would be unable to walk.

"But that was not what he told me at all. The scans had shown a tumor at the base of my neck, and the doctor said it needed to be biopsied immediately. The biopsy showed the tumor was cancerous."

"Oh, my God!" I interjected.

"Oh, no, Chaplain," Mr. Liu quickly broke in. "Fortunately, that is not the end of my story, or else I would not be here now to tell it to you.

"Because of the timing of the biopsy, the tumor was small, only in its beginning stage. That allowed the doctors to catch it and treat it early. As a result, I have been in the doctors' words 'relatively cancer-free,' since, as they have told me, the cancer can reappear at any time, and even more widespread than before. However, according to the report I just received this morning, the doctors said they cannot find any trace of the cancer at all!"

"That's great news!" I exclaimed.

"But you see, Chaplain," continued Mr. Liu, "to me, there is even better news than that.

"Had I not slipped on the stones while crossing the brook after visiting my parents' graves, I would not have suffered the injury to my neck that caused me to see my doctor in the first place. Consequently, I would never have had all those tests that eventually identified the tumor early enough to treat it and save my life. And do you know the meaning of that for me, Chaplain?"

I knew Mr. Liu didn't want or expect me to answer his question. So I just sat and waited for him to answer it himself.

"To me, everything that has occurred—from my fall on the stones in the cemetery, to the immediate tests and treatment I got upon my return here, to the fantastic report I just received this morning—*all* of that means my parents have forgiven me for any wrongdoing or acts of disrespect I may have committed as their son. It means that despite everything, they still love me. And that, Chaplain, means more to me than anything else in the world."

And who was I to gainsay Mr. Liu's interpretation of what had happened? Yes, the circumstances he had described—walking back down the hill and slipping on the stones; injuring his neck and going for the scans; finding the tumor and treating it at an early stage; all mixed with his feelings of guilt about his failings as a son—all these things could be framed as medically-explicable in the usual chain of physical cause-and-effect events. But to *insist* on that particular framework as the *only* one to properly explain Mr. Liu's experiences, thus dismissing his own explanation altogether, seems to me as "fundamentalist," as dogmatically closed to any alternative interpretation, as that of any proverbial Bible-thumper. Flatly categorizing Mr. Liu's fall as "accidental" strikes me as no more reasonable *in and of itself* than characterizing his slip as "occasioned" by his parents' forgiveness. In the end, Mr. Liu's case helped me see that my notions of "rationality" and "reasonable interpretation" had been far too narrow: they needed to include a place for *both* the purely physical *and* the more than merely physical.

As I continued my chaplaincy work, so, too, other cases continued to challenge my preconceived notions of what was "reasonable" and what was not. One case, in particular waged a full-scale, frontal assault on my previously-held notions of reason and reality.

Each day before going on rounds with the intensivist and nurses in the ICU and CCU, I would stop by the Chaplain's Office to read the computer printout indicating the patients who had requested visits. One morning, the list displayed the name "Sally Meredith"; it logged her as a Baptist. When I subsequently went up to the CCU, her chart's H&P identified her as a fifty-three-year-old, single African-American with diabetes who had been hospitalized for observation the night before, after she had arrived at the ER by ambulance following a possible heart attack.

But when I went to Ms. Meredith's room to see her, she wasn't there. Instead, I met her brother, Grady, and he, I learned, had been the one to make the request for a chaplaincy visit. A tall, imposing, dignified man, Grady told me the reason for the request.

With growing frustration in his voice, he explained, "Sally's always been head-strong and stubborn. Her pride matters a lot to her, sometimes too much for her own good, I think. Even though the doctor wants her to stay another day or two for some tests, she thinks a nurse last night disrespected her, and so now, she wants to up and go home today just as soon as she can. The doctor said that she would be leaving . . . Shoot! I can't remember the letters he used to mean she would be leaving on her own without anybody's official say-so!"

"You mean 'AMA'?" I asked. "Against Medical Advice?"

"Yeah, that's it. Anyway, I don't know what happened with the nurse last night. Lord knows, I've had a bellyful of white folks mistreating me during my lifetime. But right now, I want Sally to stay here to make sure she's OK."

Since I didn't see Sally anywhere, I assumed it was too late and that she had already packed up her things and was getting the paperwork done for her discharge. "I'm very sorry about any mistreatment your sister might have suffered last night, but I'm even sorrier I didn't get here sooner. Maybe the two of us could have persuaded her to change her mind before she decided to check herself out."

"Hold on, Chaplain! Don't get the wrong idea. Praise Jesus, I was able to talk her into waiting around long enough to have a few lab tests for her diabetes before going back home. See, I know that Sally can't stand the idea of wasting time. She thinks that's literally a sin, and what's more, I also think that deep down, she knows she has to be careful about the diabetes.

"Still, though, when she comes back from the lab, maybe she will have calmed down enough for me to talk some sense into her so that she'll stay here a while longer. Now I know you must be busy, what with all the other sick people here and such, but if I can talk her into staying, I sure would appreciate your coming back to see her and speak to her about staying for a few days more so the doctor can make sure she's fine."

"I'll tell you what, Mr. Meredith," I answered. "I'll come back again later this afternoon to visit your sister before my shift ends at five o'clock. From there, we'll just have to wait to see what happens."

"Thank you, Chaplain. I'll be praying about it," Grady responded.

The way the rest of my day went after that, I could have used any help I could get, including someone's praying *for me*. I was paged from one emergency to another. First, I had to rush down to the doors of the ER to meet parents whose only child, a nineteen-year-old college student, had arrived DOA from anaphylactic shock after having inadvertently eaten Indian food prepared with peanut oil that triggered the severe peanut allergy she had. Next, I was called to be with a patient, with whom I prayed for over two hours as he sat still stunned by his doctor having told him less than fifteen minutes before my arrival that he had an inoperable brain tumor that would likely leave him with at most three months to live, and moreover, that in the time he had left, he would probably suffer increasing delusion, blindness, and pain. Then, I was paged to another death, this time in the ICU to console an inconsolable husband whose wife of fifty years had, after lingering a few days, finally succumbed following a crash with a drunk driver.

And why page me, the chaplain, to each of these situations? The medical staff certainly didn't page me because they were callous, as though they "had better things to do." No, they called me because they simply didn't know *what* to do. As if I did. I would often marvel at how they could stand, forearms deep inside some patient's guts, feet soaked by a patient's blood, the ticking of the clock competing with the beating of the patient's heart, and still maintain their concentration, composure, and capability. But let a patient die, let a family member cry, and they seemed as helpless as the dead and their bereft survivors. So they would page me. They would call me to deal with the aftermath of tragedy, as if I had the magic words—or, on this particular day, even the time—to make it all better. But, of course, for these patients and their loved ones, no matter how much time I or anyone might have, it would never ultimately be enough to make things "all better."

Experience had taught me that lesson, and as they say, experience is a hard teacher: first she gives the test, *then* the lesson. My seminary training had tried to teach me just the opposite. As a rabbi, it was implied, I had to be the one who always knew the right thing to say. For instance, I had a pastoral psychology course whose final exam question asked the following question:

> If you were the chaplain on duty at a hospital, and a woman's husband had died in the operating room, how would you break the news to her back out in the waiting room?

Perhaps because I was a wise-ass, or maybe because even then, I knew there was no good answer, I wrote, "Ma'am, you might want to think twice about buying that new set of eighty-thousand-mile radial tires for your husband's car."

Now, some twenty years later, I knew that writing an answer like that was not a sign of being a smart-aleck, but of being smart about how dumb, how mute, I could be in the face of such life-shattering moments.

And yet, near shift's end, around 4:30, I still had one more dose of magic verbiage I was expected to dispense—words persuading Sally Meredith to stay in the hospital instead of checking herself out AMA. I went back to the CCU to find her, but couldn't. After asking around, I learned she had been moved off the unit to a room on one of the hospital's main floors, having agreed to spend the night for observation. Now at last, near the conclusion of a day filled with impossible expectations of me, I had finally gotten one I could meet by merely keeping my promise to Grady to return and visit his sister before I left for the day.

When I found the right room, Grady was sitting there in a chair next to his sister's bed. The woman showed no trace of the hostility I thought I might encounter, given what I had been told about her earlier.

"Sally," said Grady, "This is the chaplain I told you about. He came by this morning to see you when you were gone to have those tests. He promised to come back to see you later, and sure enough, here he is."

"I'm pleased to meet you, Ms. Meredith," I said, thinking that I was simply pleased to have the chance to meet her at all.

"Thank you, Chaplain," she replied warmly. "I'm mighty glad to see you, too, and you just call me Sally. That's what I've always asked my pastors to call me ever since I was a little girl. It just feels more natural and comfortable to me."

"All right then, Sally. I'm awfully glad to see you here, especially because this morning, I thought you were going to leave in spite of what your doctor thought would be best for you."

"Oh, I get that way sometimes, Chaplain. Just ornery, I guess. Grady can tell you I've been that way ever since we were kids. I don't like hospitals to begin with, and I just didn't like the way I was being treated by some nurse last night. So I got my hackles up and was ready to go, but after a while today, I realized that would just be biting off my nose to spite my face. And look, I'm out of that awful CCU in a nice quiet room, Grady's right here, and I'm feeling a lot better."

Good, I thought, no magic words from me required here. Just plain old conversation, the kind that mixes "tea and sympathy." So we talked for a time until, sneaking a look at my watch, I saw that it was already 5:30 and therefore, well past my shift's end. Consequently, as a way of wrapping things up and concluding the visit, I asked if we might all join hands in prayer, with each of us going around the circle to add some words of our own.

I can't remember who went first or last, or, for that matter, what anybody said in particular, but I vividly recall what happened when we finished.

Grady suddenly exclaimed, "Oh, that was powerful! I could feel it!"

Sally immediately joined in, "Me, too!"

And then she began to do something that at once baffled and alarmed me. Using her legs, she started pushing down the bed sheets from over her knees while simultaneously hoisting her hospital gown up over them.

"My knees hurt so, Chaplain. It's from the diabetes. Would you put your hands on them and say another prayer?" she asked. And then, almost as a proviso, she added: "And say it in Jesus' name."

I was flabbergasted—not by her request of me as a chaplain, but *as a Jew*. Ever since I was a child, all the Jews I had ever known had disparaged faith healing, the laying on of hands, as *goyisch*, as the kind of thing that only ignorant Gentiles would do or believe in. Part of the reason Jews mocked non-Jews for such beliefs is that many, if not most, Jews when sick, put their trust not in faith healing, nor in prayer, nor even in God, but in doctors, in medical science, and above all, in rationality. Thus, given my upbringing, both religious and secular, only one word fit what Sally wanted me to do: *irrational.*

And then there was the other thing Sally had asked me to do. Again, ever since childhood, I had learned that invoking, even saying, the "J-word" was anathema to Jews. Jews, from the most religious to the most assimilated, virtually gag when prayers are offered "in Jesus' name," whether at PTA meetings, Rotary luncheons, or political gatherings. I can remember, as can countless other Jews, standing as children round the piano in school during music class in December while singing one of the so-called "seasonal songs" and coming to the word, "Jesus," and at that point, *humming.*

Finally, as if all this were not enough for me to confront, Sally had placed me in a difficult position professionally. By pushing down her bed sheets and hitching up her gown and asking me to touch her uncovered knees, she had in effect asked me to venture into territory ripe with possible sexual allegations of moral misconduct, especially for a chaplain, whether Jewish or not.

Yes, her brother was present and in agreement with her. But the plain fact was that, at that moment, I was not thinking of his presence or of the risk associated with touching a female patient. Nor was I thinking about violating the shibboleth of offering a prayer in Jesus' name. Nor was I even thinking about all my reasons for dismissing the laying on hands as just plain crazy. No, instead, shocked though I was, my brain and gut could only focus on my obligation that once I'd entered a patient's room as a chaplain, everything revolved around the patient's needs rather than mine.

To be sure, I do have limits with patients' requests of me. For example, even though several hospice patients with end-stage cancer have asked me to help them obtain enough morphine to commit suicide, I have repeatedly turned down such requests to help them end their lives. For spiritual care is, after all, about keeping the spirit alive—and perhaps with it, the body as well.

Part of what kept chaplaincy alive for me entailed its constantly leading, pushing, and even dragging me to places I would otherwise never go. Had I, for instance, known ahead of time any or all of what Sally would ask me to do, I may well have sent another chaplain in my stead, a black Christian woman perhaps. But I had promised Grady to come back to see Sally before leaving for the day, and now his sister and he had asked for the kind of spiritual support I had no right to deny them. Once I had come through the threshold of Sally's hospital room, I had left behind the familiar borders of my own spiritual homeland.

I put my hands on Sally's bare knees. Grady took Sally's hands in his. And as though speaking through a voice not my own, I said, "God of all flesh, you surely know how Sally suffers. You surely feel the pain in her knees as much as she does. Therefore, Lord, please relieve her pain, take it away, and replace it with comfort and ease. We ask all this in Jesus' name."

"Amen!" said Sally. "That was *so* powerful. I could really feel it."

"Me, too!" Grady quickly added.

Sally followed just as quickly, saying, "I feel less pain already, Chaplain. Thank you so much."

Taking a deep breath of relief (and hoping there would be no more requests by either of them), I responded matter-of-factly, "No need for thanks. I'm glad I could be of help."

After making the customary pleasantries to say good-bye—including getting Sally's assurance that she would not leave the hospital until the medical staff thought it proper for her to go home—I turned to go. Then, as I went through the doorway of her room, a chill went up my spine. I didn't think much of it except its likely reflecting some kind of release of the tension that the laying on of hands and all that went with it had just caused me.

That night, I was repeatedly awakened by terrible shooting pains in my knees.

The next day, I went to speak with my supervisor, Caryn, about what had occurred the day before. I needed to check in with her not only about the propriety of my physically touching a patient, but also perhaps, if I could bring myself to do it, about what had physically "laid hands" on me the previous night.

Caryn, a white, middle-aged woman, had years of experience and training as a hospital chaplain; an ordained minister of the United Church of Christ, she was liberal and well-educated. Yet her childhood and adolescence would hardly have served as predictors for her life to follow. She hailed from a small town in the rural Midwest, at whose core was a community almost uniformly Protestant, evangelical, and "Bible-believing."

In such a place, questioning and probing evoked suspicion rather than praise.

I began by telling Caryn about my having touched Sally's knees along, of course, with the reason I had done it. I purposely didn't mention the part about praying in Jesus' name. That part of the story still made me feel uncomfortable, and besides, although Caryn might "outrank" me as a chaplain, I was the one with the PhD in systematic theology—*and* a circumcised penis. Caryn nevertheless reassured me that in placing my hands on Sally's knees, I had done nothing wrong.

She wasn't through, though, with what she had to tell me. "I don't know if I ever shared this with you," Caryn continued, "but my grandfather was much respected as a faith healer in the place where I grew up. People would come from all around to have him lay hands on them to help them with various physical ailments they might have."

"Now," I thought to myself, "she's going to tell me about how the mere psychological 'power of suggestion' can at times help people, and that's what had happened when I had placed my hands on Sally's knees."

But Caryn didn't explain it that way at all, and by not doing so, she didn't try to explain it away.

"Once, when I was about sixteen or seventeen, they brought my grandfather a woman who had been in a serious farm accident and who was hemorrhaging badly from a large, deep gash in her stomach. Although a doctor had been sent for, he was miles away in some other part of the county, and meanwhile, no one could stop the bleeding from the woman's belly. So although she and her family certainly believed in and used modern medicine, they knew my grandfather's reputation and without anywhere else to turn, they put their trust in him and in his purported healing powers. The woman's family brought her into my grandparents' house and laid her down on the kitchen table, and then I watched as my grandfather took his hands and placed—not *pressed*, but placed—them on the woman's abdomen and offered prayer, and then suddenly, the hemorrhaging stopped."

Then Caryn paused and asked me something I thought quite odd. "Michael, after you finished laying your hands on the lady's knees and saying a prayer, did you feel anything strange?"

I thought back to what happened after I said goodbye to Sally and Grady. "Just as I was about to leave the room, there was a shiver in my spine. I wrote it off to the emotional intensity and the nervous energy of the whole experience for me."

Caryn looked straight into my eyes and asked, "Did the shiver go from top down, or from bottom up?"

I had never bothered to think about it until then. What difference did it make anyway? "It went from the base of my spine up to my neck."

"That's the way it would go for my grandfather, too. You see, for most people, shivers go from the top down."

I didn't know what to say. What on earth could possibly count as a sensible response? Did I have a power that I didn't know of? Could I help other people by placing my hands on them while praying for them? Had I failed other people by *not* doing that? And had my closing the prayer "in Jesus' name" been the key for making it "work"? But perhaps most troubling to me as a Jew—*as a rabbi!*—was my invoking Jesus' name in the first place, whether it worked or not.

I called my doctoral dissertation director and mentor, Thad, an internationally-recognized Christian theologian, and told him about my misgivings. As always, he spoke softly and slowly and only after having first taken several moments to reflect on his response.

"Michael," he said, "Some people think that to pray 'in Jesus' name' is like talking to God through some kind of supernatural pipeline. But to pray in Jesus' name really means to pray with a character, with a disposition, like Jesus', that is, to talk to and with God *humbly*."

Thad knew what he was talking about. In the TaNaKH, the Hebrew Bible, peoples' names are not arbitrary monikers attached to them. Instead, their names personify their character, or in other words, who at bottom they *are*. For instance, the name of the Biblical patriarch, Jacob, derives from a root meaning "heel." And, at least for the first part of his life, the name says almost everything there is to say about him as a human being. At birth, he tries to grab the heel of his twin brother, Esau, thus usurping Esau's place—and prerogatives—as first to emerge from their mother's womb. Growing up, he continues to act as a "heel" by cheating his brother out of the blessing due the first born by deceiving their blind father, Isaac, on Isaac's deathbed. Not until much later, after Jacob wrestles with a being who divinely blesses him with a name change—*Israel*—does his character, his name in the world, change for the better. Even nowadays, we, too, equate "having a good name" with someone's *having character*. So in praying to God "in Jesus' name," by sacrificing as it were my own feelings and beliefs on Sally's behalf, I had crossed no line. Had that kind of sacrifice for others not been precisely what Jesus had made, too?

Of course, there was another part of Jesus' self-sacrifice as well: the pain he endured on others' behalf.

By chance, a few days later I had to visit my attorney on some business. Her name was Tanya, and she was an African-American transplant to the Bay Area from Louisiana. When I went into her office, she noticed I was limping a little.

"What happened to you? Forget that you're middle-aged and try to play some hoops with the kids?"

"No, not at all," I answered.

"Well, why are you a little gimpy then?"

It was one thing to tell my supervisor about my experience with Sally, another to talk about it with Thad, but talking with a hard-nosed lawyer like Tanya about it was something else again.

"This may take some time and sound a little strange. You sure you want to hear it?" I asked. Now *I* felt like the patient worried about the chaplain's open-mindedness.

"Go ahead, I'm all ears!" she said. "Consider the billable hour clock turned off."

I told her the whole story, ending with the night the pain in my knees kept me awake.

When I finished, Tanya leaned forward in her chair, coming within a few inches of my face and said in a very quiet voice, "The spirits were kind to you, on account of your being new at this."

"*The what?!*" I stammered.

"Now lookie here," Tanya explained. "You know I grew up in Louisiana. Well, I knew folks who did this all the time. Sure, there were some who claimed to have the gift and didn't. But there were others who sure as hell did have it. I saw it for myself.

"Let me ask you a question, though," she continued. "Were you grounded when you put your hands on that woman?"

"What do you mean 'grounded'?"

"Were you touching anything besides the woman's knees? Did you have one hand on something else like a table, or better yet, in some water?"

"No. I had both my hands on her knees."

"That's why the pain went from her knees into *yours*. It had no place else to go to." Tanya spoke as if she were giving a summation to a jury. "And that's why the spirits were pretty kind to you. They knew this was your first time."

Now I didn't know what to think. The laying on of hands, Jesus' name, spirits—all this was entirely beyond my prior way of thinking about the world and how it functioned. And while I've certainly touched people since then—hugging them, for example, or holding their hands to comfort them—I've never since tried to heal them by placing my hands on them and praying to God "in Jesus' name" to take away their affliction while using me as a vehicle. Maybe I haven't done it because it's too frightening for me to believe it—to think that God might actually use me that way. Or maybe I haven't done it because despite what I experienced first-hand with Sally, I still don't believe it myself.

But one thing I do believe from my experience with Mr. Liu and Sally. Mysteries surround healing that cannot be reduced to clinical science *alone*. For if you have ever sat by the bedside of someone who was breathing one moment and then not breathing the next, you know somewhere deep inside you that the mystery of life, the mystery of our very existence, remains just that.

4

Jenny's Hand

A S THE ICU TEAM made its morning rounds through the horseshoe of patient cubicles, the doctor leading it stopped at the bed of an old woman who lay sleeping. He stretched out his arm, flattened his palm, and traced an arc slowly downward.

Although Dr. Booth was an unassuming man, given neither to histrionics nor hyperbole, his gesture underscored both the graveness of the case and the gravity of his title: "Intensivist." He gazed down at the patient's chart and made a note. When he finally spoke, his voice was barely audible.

"This lady is Mrs. Jenny Lubinsky, she is eighty-four, and she has congestive heart failure. She was admitted last night after having had a possible MI.[1] Although she's stabilized for now, her decline, though gradual, is inevitable. If she goes into full cardiac arrest, we won't be able to bring her back. Her bones are so brittle, they'll crumble if we put the paddles on her."[2]

Dr. Booth's speaking first on rounds about a patient was, for him, unprecedented. Typically, the patient's nurse would open any discussion by reporting what had happened the shift before. Then any other team members would have their say—therapists and techs of various sorts going first, social worker and chaplain chipping in afterwards—with Dr. Booth generally the last to take a turn. Yet the old woman's very presence in the ICU represented a reversal of its natural order. Normally, the ICU was the initial stop for the deathly-ill on the road to recovery. But from what Dr. Booth had done and said, it seemed that for Jenny Lubinksy,

---

1. That is, a myocardial infarction, or less technically, a heart attack.
2. I.e., defibrillator paddles.

the ICU would be little more than a way station on an unalterable course toward death.

As soon as rounding ended thirty minutes later (neither patients nor staff could afford any more time away from one another than that), I made my way back to Mrs. Lubinksky's bed. From what I had heard earlier, I thought she might appreciate a visit. I needed to try to make sure, though, and the chart, as always, provided a good starting point. I skimmed down to the box, "Decline Chaplaincy Visit" and saw it had no checkmark. But that wasn't necessarily enough to warrant I would be welcome. ER personnel, especially during a crisis "admit" such as Mrs. Lubinsky's, frequently failed to record a patient's religious preferences accurately, if at all. However, notations a little farther down the page showed me that in this instance, someone in the ER had taken the time to try to get things right. Under "Religion," a checkmark abutted "Jewish," followed by the entry: "Pt. belongs to Temple Emmanuel. Rabbi is Charles Lifkin." I knew both her synagogue—it was one of the largest Reform temples in the area—and its rabbi. If I accomplished nothing else during my visit, I could at least offer to call him to drop by and see her.

I put the chart back down, walked over to her cubicle, and knocked on its frame. "Hello, Mrs. Lubinsky, I'm Rabbi Michael Goldberg," I said, getting to introduce myself in a way rare for me since I generally had so few Jewish patients. "I'm a chaplain on the hospital staff. Would you like me to stop by and see you while you're here?"

"*Nu?*" she replied, "So what are you doing now?"

I took that as a "Yes."

"So what's going on?" I asked.

"So you tell me. Do I look like I'm the one who has seen my chart today?" she answered with a grin.

Some might have found Mrs. Lubinsky's rejoinder quite unnerving if not off-putting altogether. But to me, it was inviting and reassuring, a piece of the jesting repartee that constitutes good old-fashioned Jewish *schmoozing*. Sometimes, in fact, a Jewish patient's very welfare may hinge on a medical professional's ability to *schmooze*.

I once got paged to a patient's room by a neurophysiologist. When I arrived, the doctor pointed to a plump, elderly woman and whispered, "I think this lady has dementia."

"What makes you think that?" I asked, having no idea why I, a chaplain, had been summoned to the bedside in such circumstances.

The neurophysiologist merely replied, "Go ahead; just talk to her."

I went over to the patient and said by way of introduction, "Hello, my name is Michael. I'm a chaplain. The doctor asked me to stop by. How are you doing today?"

"So how should I be doing?" she responded.

"I don't know. Why don't you tell me what's been going on?"

"What's to tell? It's a hospital, right?"

"You're absolutely right. It *is* a hospital. But I guess like most patients here, you'd rather be home."

Wryly—and with perfect timing—the woman answered, "So the service here is a little better, maybe?"

"See?!" the neurophysiologist broke in. "Every time I ask her a question, she only answers with another question!" Then, sheepishly, the physician added, "I've heard that's what Jews do."

I took a look at the lady's chart. She *was* Jewish, having come to the United States from Eastern Europe right before the Holocaust. I confirmed for the doctor's benefit that such banter back-and-forth is indeed what Jews (often) do, and that moreover, its absence in a Jewish patient might indicate the presence of depression. Were it not for my "specialist consult," the neurophysiologist might have diagnosed her patient's *schmoozing* as dementia. *Oy.*

Knowing how to *schmooze* is no less critical for chaplains than it is for other practitioners when it comes to serving Jewish patients. Initially entering a Jewish patient's room and saying "I'm Chaplain So-and-So from the Spiritual Care Department" is a almost a sure-fire way to be immediately asked to leave. The very words "chaplain" and "spiritual" are simply not within most Jews' realm of discourse. Those words come from a Christian lexicon, many of whose terms, such as "Christ" and "conversion," carry connotations that for Jews are historically horrific. Nor can any chaplain—even a Jewish one—walk into a Jewish patient's room and assume that God will be part of any ensuing conversation. According to the latest study of American Jews, fewer than forty percent belong to synagogues while an even smaller percentage participate in any religious practice more regular than the yearly observance of the Passover Seder, Channukkah, or Yom Kippur.[3] Thus, the good-natured give-and-take of

3. Mandel L. Berman and Edward H. Kaplan, Co-Chairs, *National Jewish Population Survey 2000–2001* (New York: United Jewish Communities, 2001) 7.

schmoozing, with its circuitous course of chitchat, may provide one of the safest and most fruitful ways of starting a conversation with Jewish patients. At some point, it may just put them enough at ease to begin talking about what matters most—their illness, their fears, even God.

Even short of those things, though, family frequently affords an easy entry point for *schmoozing*, and I had learned from Mrs. Lubinsky's chart that she had two daughters. I suspected I wouldn't have to do much prodding to get her to *schmooze* a little about them with me.

"Mrs. Lubinsky, besides your doctors, nurses and me, has anybody else come by today—friends or family, for example?"

"First, Rabbi, call me Jenny; it already feels cold enough in here as it is. Anyway, I have two daughters. My older one, Lois, called me a little while ago. She's an office manager for a large company in the city. Such a smart, competent girl! Always has been! Her sister, Debbie, is a second-grade teacher near where I live, and she's supposed to stop by later. She has such a way with the children she teaches. In a way, she's very childlike herself; maybe that's why she understands her little ones so well. Any way you put it, I'm very lucky to have two such wonderful children." Then, all of a sudden, her voice faltered. "My girls are particularly important to me now that my husband is gone. He died three months ago."

I could have followed up and asked her about her husband's death. But I didn't know her well enough yet to presume to enter into so intimate a territory. Before leaving, though, and notwithstanding the aforementioned widespread American Jewish aversion to traditional religious practices, I at least wanted to offer to say a prayer.

"Jenny," I inquired, "would you like me to recite a *MiSheBerach*[4] for you?"

"Look, Rabbi," she said with a little smile, "I know I'm sick. But I'm not *that* sick."

"That's fine; I understand," I said, "but would you like me to call your synagogue and have Rabbi Lifkin come visit you?"

Again, she demurred. "No, he's already so busy. I don't want to bother him."

Since she had now declined a visit from her own rabbi, I wondered if she would likewise turn down another one from me.

---

4. Hebrew for "May the One who blessed"; these are the opening words of the traditional prayer asking for God's healing of the sick.

"Well, then, would you mind if I dropped in on you some other time?"

Like a veteran Catskills comic delivering a can't-miss comeback line, she looked at me and, without missing a beat, replied: "Well, it couldn't hurt."

Later that afternoon, I had to return to the ICU to see another patient. On my way out, I spied a slender, curly-haired woman sitting at Jenny's bedside. As I walked past, Jenny spotted me out of the corner of her eye.

"Debbie, there's the chaplain I mentioned to you. Rabbi, do you have a moment? Who would have thought they would have a rabbi in this place?"

"Rabbi," began Debbie, "I'm so glad you're here to be with Mom."

As I got closer, I could see that Debbie had been crying. She looked wan and haggard. "Debbie, I'm glad to meet you. How does your mother seem this afternoon?"

"She seems better than when I saw her last night in the emergency room." Then Debbie turned toward me enough to block Jenny's direct line of sight. Keeping her right hand slightly below her waist, she signaled toward the ICU's open area beyond her mother's cubicle.

I tried not to give her away. After making some small talk for a few more minutes, I started to take my leave. "Well, I have some other visits to make this afternoon before I go home for *Shabbat*. I hope you two can have, as much as possible under the circumstances, a *Shabbat Shalom*.[5] I'll be back in the hospital Sunday, Jenny. If you're still a guest here in one of our spacious suites and you'd like to see me, just have them page me to come by."

"*Shabbat Shalom* to you, too, Rabbi," said Jenny. "I appreciate your offer. I just might take you up on it."

I started to leave when Debbie, now playing *her* part in our little one-act, interjected, "Oh, Rabbi, you made me think of something one of my kids brought up in class today. Mom, why don't you try to rest? I'll be right back."

"Take your time, Dear."

Debbie and I moved a few steps out on to the floor, away from Jenny's cubicle.

---

5. I.e., a "peaceful Sabbath."

"Rabbi," she began, "I know my mother is seriously ill. But this is so hard. We just lost our father a little while ago, and I don't know how we can handle another death. We're still in shock over Dad's. He just had a sudden heart attack. Unlike Mom, he had never even had any previous heart problems.

"Our family physician, Dr. Greenfield, has taken care of us all for years, but he doesn't seem able to give us any guidance. We've even turned to Rabbi Lifkin, who has been our rabbi since we were children at the temple. While Rabbi Lifkin has been very nice, he doesn't seem to be able to give us any more direction than Dr. Greenfield."

"What kind of advice are you looking for from them?" I asked.

"I don't know," Debbie whimpered. "But if I want to talk more with you, may I?"

"Of course," I said. And with that, Debbie turned and walked back to her mother.

I returned to the hospital on Sunday. There were no rounds on weekends. But there was a note for me in the office that Jenny wanted to see me. I took the elevator up the four floors to the ICU, acknowledged the stoic and not-so-stoic family members in its waiting room, and entered the hospital's Holy of Holies, a solemn place filled with both hope and dread.

As I walked past her station, Charlene, the charge nurse, called me over. "Look out over there for Mrs. Lubinsky's older daughter, Lois," she said, motioning toward a tall, angular woman standing over Jenny's bed. "The chart lists her as the primary caregiver, but she just refuses to get with the program. Neither Dr. Booth nor even their family doc, Greenfield, can get her to face what's happening."

Across the floor, Jenny had already caught sight of me. Waving me over, she skipped the customary introductions for the kind far more favored by proud Jewish mothers through the ages: "Rabbi, this is my Lois, my oldest and wisest girl. I simply don't know what I'd do without her!"

Frostily, Lois muttered, "Hello, Rabbi."

Undaunted, I replied, "It's good to meet you, Lois. Your mother mentioned you when she was telling me the other day what wonderful children she has. Today, when I arrived at the office, I found a message from her asking me to come by again."

Consciously now directing the discussion away from Lois and back to Jenny, I said, "So what can I do for you?"

"Well, Rabbi, it's like you said just now. I'm so lucky to have such fine girls who have been so good about coming to see me. But the doctors? *Feh*! They haven't been so good about dropping by. I haven't really seen any of them since Friday. Who knows? Maybe they take the weekend off? Anyway, what do you think they plan to do with me?"

"Jenny," I replied, "I'm no Maimonides—no rabbi and doctor combined in one! I don't know anything more about your condition medically than you, probably less. Even if I could understand the chart notes your doctors and nurses have left, I wouldn't be allowed to share them with you, because I'm neither medically trained nor certified to do so. Consequently, I'm afraid I really don't have any medical updates to give you. But maybe you or Lois could update me about what's been going on since I saw you Friday."

"Just visiting with my mother," Lois said in a voice that was, if possible, even more unfriendly than before.

"The rabbi can figure that out, Lois," Jenny chided her. "Tell him what we've been talking about."

Barely looking over at me, Lois "volunteered" a bit more information: "We've all known for a while that Mother has congestive heart disease. When she had a lot of trouble breathing Thursday night, we rushed her to the emergency room. What we want to know is what can be done to make her better."

Only a while ago, Jenny had paid Lois the compliment of referring to her as her "wisest girl." But Lois at present seemed anything but astute when it came to her mother's prognosis. And who could blame her for her apparent lack of insight? She had recently lost one parent. How could she bear the loss of the other? Without doubt, Debbie also shared in the suffering stemming from their mother's decline. Yet to Lois, the conscientious elder child to whom primary caregiver responsibility had fallen, a double measure of misery may well have been apportioned.

Abruptly, Lois turned toward me and curtly said, "Mother appreciated your coming by." Not "I've appreciated your coming by," much less "I'd appreciate your coming by again." As far as Lois was concerned, if I didn't have any positive news about the doctors' plan of care for Jenny, I had nothing of any value to offer, nor, for that matter, did anyone who didn't know how "to make her better." Taken aback and by surprise, I awkwardly made my goodbyes.

Because I worked Sunday, I got Monday off. By the time I returned to work on Tuesday, Jenny's condition had worsened considerably. She lay connected to a ventilator, a plastic tube jutting from her mouth. An ER nurse once told me that were she herself ever found unconscious in a car wreck, she wanted "Do Not Intubate!" tattooed across her chest. "I don't want a tube snaked down my throat," she said emphatically, before adding every bit as forcefully, "and who the hell can say when they'll ever be able to take the damn thing out?!" As for Jenny, whatever purchase on oxygen the tube's insertion might have gained her had come at a steep cost: her ability to speak. Hadn't her capacity to *schmooze*, after all, gotten her companionship and commiseration even amidst the isolation of the ICU? With the tube having stifled Jenny's chief means of agency, I wondered if it had reduced her to a patient in the word's most basic sense: a mere sufferer incapable of anything but enduring without complaint.

I didn't need to wait long to get an answer. Later that afternoon as I was walking the hall between the ICU and the CCU, I came across Beth, the social worker on the floor. She grabbed me by the elbow and walked me over toward the hallway windows facing onto the Bay as though to find a more private setting, out of the flow of the foot traffic of staff and visitors bustling through the corridor.

"After rounds this morning," she whispered, "I had to go back to the ICU to look for something I thought I had left there. As long as I was there, I thought I'd look in on Mrs. Lubinsky again. We all know how hard intubation can be. Anyway, from the moment I sat down, she kept shifting her eyes over toward her bed stand. I finally realized she wanted the pad and pencil lying on it. When I gave them to her, she took them and after lots of effort managed to scrawl out, 'I want to die! Take out the tube!'"

Although I was shocked by what Beth had just told me, I was even more stunned that she would tell me, of all people, in the first place. She was always professionally civil to me, but hardly warm. An avowedly secular Jew, if Beth believed in any scripture, it was *The Diagnostic and Statistical Manual of Mental Disorders*, 4th edition. Known in the trade as "The DSM IV," it lumps religious and spiritual problems with "other conditions that may be a focus of clinical attention."[6] From Beth's perspective, such clinical attention, if required, was to be given by social workers, psy-

6. American Psychiatric Association, *Diagnostic and Statistical Manual of Mental Disorders*, 4th ed. (Washington, DC: American Psychiatric Association, 1994) §V62.89, 685.

chologists, or psychiatrists—*not*, in other words, by chaplains. In her eyes, having a chaplain care for a patient's religious or spiritual problems was tantamount to treating the symptom with more of the disease. Why, then, had she come to me to talk about what had transpired with Jenny?

Caught off guard at least as much by Beth's actions in approaching me as by anything Jenny might have done, I blurted out, "Well, what did you do, Beth?"

"What *could* I do?" Beth replied in a voice filled with equal parts anguish and agitation. "I charted it, of course. And then I called Lois. And do you know what she did? She called for a psychiatric consult! So Dr. Anderson came by and prescribed Prozac for depression!"

"He *what*?" I exclaimed, mirroring Beth's own distress. "What could possibly be more normal for somebody in Mrs. Lubinsky's circumstances than to feel depressed?"

"Exactly!" Beth answered indignantly. "And I'm really upset that Anderson went to anti-depressants as a first resort when everybody knows how hard it is to use them effectively with patients who are Mrs. Lubinsky's age!" Now I understood why Beth had come to me instead of to a nurse or even to a fellow social work to express her alarm. Precisely because she didn't count me as part of the multi-disciplinary team, she reckoned me as "safe."

By this point, Beth was so irate, she could hardly contain herself. "But you know what's the worst thing of all concerning Mrs. Lubinsky's treatment? It's the way she's being treated by Lois. That daughter of hers just doesn't seem to care at all about what her mother wants—or needs!" And then Beth turned around and briskly walked away, back down the corridor to go on about her business. Apparently, she felt she had said to me all she needed to.

For the next three days on rounds, I listened eagerly to hear whether Jenny's physical or emotional condition had improved. Each day, how-ever, the report remained the same: unchanged. After rounds the third day, I decided to see Jenny for myself and learn what I could first-hand. When I entered her cubicle, I found her dozing lightly.

"Jenny," I said softly, "It's Rabbi Goldberg."

She slowly opened her eyes and took a few moments to focus.

When I felt sure she was alert, I continued, "I thought you might be able to use some company. I can't begin to imagine how you must feel right now. But I want you to know that I'm glad to see you and to do whatever I can for you."

A tear rolled down her cheek. Then, without warning, she started glancing over at her bedstand—and at the pad and pencil. Uneasily, I handed them to her. She took the pencil in her quivering hand, pressed down hard on the paper, and finally scribbled out, "Take out the tube! I want to die! Tell Debbie!"

I fear the day when hospitals might routinely comply with requests such as Jenny's. My apprehensiveness springs in part from my religious belief that our lives are not our own, that they do not simply belong to us by right but come to us as gifts and trusts. Much more, however, my trepidation stems from the prospect of hospitals or HMOs employing on their staffs Kevorkian-like specialists who offer a procedure termed not "physician-assisted suicide" (an oxymoron if ever there were one), but "medicide," a practice touted as a low-cost, compassionate way of ending "pointless" suffering. And yet for all my reservations regarding Jenny's wishes, I had absolutely no qualms about at least voicing them to Debbie. For were I to have ignored her by responding to her as did Lois and Dr. Anderson, the psychiatrist, I would have been treating her as if she were a helpless mute, if not, in fact, as already dead. I took the note from Jenny and promised her, "I'll make sure this gets to Debbie."

I sat silently by her bed for a few more minutes. Previously, when I had asked her whether she would like me to say a prayer for her, she had joked that she was "not *that* sick." Now she was.

"Jenny, would you like a *MiSheBerach*?" I offered.

She just looked away.

"That's fine, Jenny. I'm still glad to come by and visit and try to help you to the best of my ability."

After I left, I thought about calling Debbie right away. In the end, though, I decided against it. I certainly wasn't going to have a chat over the phone about such an emotionally fraught subject, nor, for that matter, did I intend to give Debbie the time to call Lois to accompany her and thereby sabotage Jenny's request that I speak to Debbie specifically. I chose instead to have the ICU staff page me the next time they saw Debbie on the floor.

The page came later that afternoon. I met Debbie in the ICU waiting room and asked her if I could have a word.

"Oh, my God, Rabbi! Has something happened with Mom?" she exclaimed.

"No, Debbie. Nothing's changed. Things are exactly where they were before."

I reached into my pocket, took out her mother's note, unfolded it, and handed it to her.

Debbie read it and began to sob. "Rabbi, how can we allow this? Isn't it suicide?! Isn't it against Jewish law?!"

Debbie's question, put by a Reform Jew for whom Jewish law had little or no authority, may have seemed to some bizarre. But coming from a distraught child clinging desperately to her dying mother, it struck me as making perfect sense. Even so, I needed to speak to the theological issues before the psychological ones, if for no other reason than, apart from my religious role at the hospital, Debbie and I would likely have never had occasion even to meet one another, let alone discuss an issue of such looming consequence.

"Debbie," I began, "like many other issues in Jewish law, there's no simple black and white when it comes to removing someone from a ventilator. Some rabbis have decided to forbid it while others have decided to permit it. Just as with American law, factors such as the patient's prognosis and mental capacity count heavily in making the decision. That said, though, there's still one decision that only you can make."

I paused some moments before proceeding; I wanted to give Debbie a chance to take in what I had just said—as well as what I was going to say next.

"Awhile ago, a veteran chaplain told me something I've never forgotten. He said that, from his experience, whenever there's a patient in a bed, there are usually other patients at the bedside who are completely unaware that they are patients, too. That's because they're so focused on giving support to the patient in the bed, they don't realize how much support they themselves need. To make matters worse, they sometimes confuse their own suffering with the sick person's and fail to see that alleviating one may not alleviate the other. Your mother has identified the source of her suffering and decided, rightly or wrongly, what she wants to do to relieve it. But that still leaves you, Debbie. What about *your* suffering?"

She started weeping. "I don't know what to do, Rabbi. First, losing Dad, and now so soon after that, Mom. . . . I just don't know what to do, Rabbi. I just don't know how to let Mom go."

"No one does, Debbie. But I do know that at the very least the *mitz-vah*[7] of honoring parents requires taking your mother's own sense of her life into account. While Judaism doesn't believe that any of us gets the ultimate say-so in what happens to us, it nonetheless insists that each of us still gets to have, so far as possible, some significant voice in our life's direction."

Debbie took some Kleenex from her purse and wiped her eyes. "Thank you, Rabbi. I've trusted Mom's judgment my whole life. I guess now, of all times, is not the time to stop. I hope Lois will feel that way, too. I'll speak with her as soon as I get home."

Feeling relieved about having kept my promise to Jenny and hopeful after my talk with Debbie, I finished up the rest of my visits for the day. I returned to the chaplain's office and was completing some paperwork before going home when the phone rang.

"Hello, Chaplain's Office, Michael Goldberg speaking."

"Rabbi Goldberg, this is Lois," said a voice so chilly it made me shiver.

Trying to compensate for Lois's coldness, I made an effort to make my voice sound as warm as possible. "Oh, hello, Lois, what can I do for you?"

The voice at the other end remained as icy as before. "Nothing, *absolutely* nothing. Debbie called me after your talk with her, and we don't want you to talk to anybody in our family anymore—especially not to Mother."

Whereas a moment before I had been feigning warmth, now I was genuinely hot. Lois could no more bar me from speaking to her mother than to her sister. Lois's gall, her sheer *chutzpah*, seemed to know no bounds! Hadn't the breathing tube itself proved enough of a bar to Jenny and me talking with each other?

Then I caught myself. I recalled what I had said to Debbie only a few hours earlier about the importance of distinguishing between one's own suffering and that of others. Unlike Jenny, I wasn't the one dying with a tube down my windpipe. Nor, unlike Lois or Debbie, was I the one about to lose my sole surviving parent. No, I was simply a staff member unlucky enough to have fielded a phone call from an irritated family member. Coming to that recognition didn't make Lois's words sting any less, but

7. Literally, "commandment"; derivatively, "good deed."

it did put them—and my own chagrin—into clearer, more manageable perspective.

"I'm sorry, Lois," I said. "I truly didn't mean to make things harder. I was only..."

Before I could say anything else, Lois cut me off. "Goodbye, Rabbi," she said flatly. Then she hung up.

I *was* sorry for Lois. Given the inevitable course of her mother's decline, her burden was not likely to be lessened, and I certainly did not intend to make it any heavier. But neither would I let her add to Jenny's suffering by keeping me away from a bedside where I had always previously been welcome. Nor, for that matter, would I hesitate to see Debbie again. I was not about to anoint Lois the "Czarina of Suffering," whose diktats decreed how everyone else would grieve in her ever-expanding empire of lament. Such emotional imperialism only falsifies the essential character of suffering, which for all its distinctive cultural manifestations,[8] nonetheless remains, if anything does, singularly subjective. Or, as Prov 14:10 more succinctly puts it, "The heart knows its own bitterness."

Despite my resolve to continue seeing Jenny and Debbie, circumstances throughout the next week prevented me from talking to either one. Jenny was always asleep or heavily medicated when I passed by her bed while Debbie, although visiting regularly according to the nurses, was always absent during my routine walks through the ICU. Meanwhile, each day during rounds, I kept recalling the very first time I had seen Jenny and watched the slow downward arc of Dr. Booth's hand. Within the amphitheater of beds forming the ICU, that gesture increasingly reminded me of the Roman arena's thumbs-down whereby some wretch was condemned to an awful end. Jenny's fate rested, though, with no capricious Caesar. It lay instead with an unbudging triumvirate of disease, technology, and family.

Finally one day on rounds, Chuck, the respiratory therapist, said aloud what individual team members had been saying privately to one another for some time. "She's just getting weaker. I doubt we'll ever be able to wean her off the vent now."

---

8. See, e.g., Mark Zborowski, *People in Pain* (San Francisco: Jossey-Bass, 1969) and the previously cited Juliene G. Lipson, Suzanne L. Dibble, Pamela A Minarik, eds., *Culture and Nursing Care* (San Francisco: UCSF Nursing Press, 1996) which sketch how different ethnic, racial, and religious groups manifest and manage suffering.

"I agree," replied Dr. Booth quietly. "And yet, if we have no real hope of helping her, she can't just stay here in the ICU, let alone at the hospital."

"You're right," Beth chimed in. "But the family, particularly Lois, will have a fit if we try to move her. We're probably going to need to have a family conference with all of us present, including the family's physician, Dr. Greenfield, and Clarice from Risk Management, too."

When the family conference was held a few days later back at Jenny's bed, I was summoned to attend; despite Lois's animus toward me (an antipathy for all I knew, now shared by Debbie as well), Risk Management had insisted on my presence. Like Beth, I, too, had charted Jenny's wish to have the vent removed, and once written down in a patient's chart, an event could not simply be "erased." Nevertheless, from the conference's outset, what Jenny wanted seemed to be the last thing that mattered.

"I don't know what we're doing here!" growled Lois as though she meant to end the meeting before it ever had a chance to begin.

Dr. Greenfield turned toward Lois and spoke, his voice low and soft, as if he were talking once again to her as a little girl in his office, "Why, Lois, we're here to help decide on a plan that's best for your mother. That's what we all want, isn't it?"

"I don't think that's what *they* want," snarled Lois, glaring at Beth, me, and the other staff. "They just want to clear a hospital bed."

"No, Lois," said Dr. Greenfield calmly," I've known this hospital and the people here for decades. They're interested only in your mother's welfare. It's just that right now, it's difficult to decide what *is* best for her." Realizing the opening he had created, he turned and said to Dr. Booth and Chuck, "What do the two of you think?"

Dr. Booth answered, "I think she's in a tough place. I doubt we'll ever be able to wean her off the vent." Chuck nodded his agreement.

If they were hoping that Lois would at last acknowledge that her mother's condition was indeed terminal and that further aggressive treatment through the vent or some other means was futile, Lois quickly disabused them.

"Well, then, we'll just have to wait and see."

And then there was silence. I kept waiting for someone—Dr. Greenfield perhaps, among those assembled the longest-known and longest-trusted—to say to the daughters, "Lois, Debbie, waiting won't help. With or without the ventilator, your mother is dying. With the vent, it will only be harder and more uncomfortable for her to die. She knows that, and she's told us that she wants the tube removed. As her children, you ought to support her decision."

But Dr. Greenfield uttered no such words. Like the rest of us—Dr. Booth, Chuck, Beth, and myself—he stood by silently. Lois's words, it turned out, were the last ones spoken by anyone there. The "conference" was over. It had lasted less than ten minutes. Making sure her sister was close behind her, Lois promptly turned to leave. As Debbie passed by me, she looked away and mumbled beneath her breath, "I'm sorry, Rabbi."

I walked away from the meeting tremendously upset. But with whom? With Lois for so imperiously squelching yet once more any voice different from her own? With Chuck and the two physicians for not being more vocal about Jenny's prognosis? With Beth for not voicing yet again Jenny's written wish to have the tube removed?

In the end, my own failure to speak up was what upset me most. Neither Lois's belligerence nor the hospital's pecking order—doctors at the top, chaplains at the bottom—truly explains my silence. I recognize, in retrospect, that I failed to speak, not because I lacked the nerve, but because I lacked the vocabulary.

The word, "hospice," for example, was not truly part of my lexicon, any more than it is in the argot of the ICU, where "care" means "cure" much more than "comfort." Intensive Care Units approach disease the way that generals go to war. No matter how "humane" they profess to be, no matter how much they talk about "supporting a patient's quality of life," in their "battle" against disease, they typically marshal whatever equipment they can muster.[9] Once that equipment, whether breathing tube or feeding tube or some other such apparatus, has been deployed, its redeployment—i.e., its removal—may become difficult if not impossible for reasons more psychological than ethical or legal. What general, after all, wants to order retreat, much less surrender?

But even if I had been able to articulate such things at Jenny's care conference, I doubt my saying them would have altered the outcome. Lois's stubbornness, combined with the culture of the ICU, made too strong a team for me to overcome. All the same, I felt draped by feelings of inadequacy in my failure to ease Jenny's suffering. So I did the only thing I could think to do. Though I was neither Jenny's family, nor a physician at whose directive the tube might be removed, I was still her chaplain,

9. See Sharon R. Kaufman, *And A Time To Die: How American Hospitals Shape the End of Life* (New York: Simon & Shuster, 2005).

through whose visit some solace might enter an otherwise insufferable situation.

When I arrived later that day to see Jenny, she was, for once, wide awake. Leaning over the bedrail, I looked down into her gray eyes, and said, "Hello, Jenny, it's Rabbi Goldberg." I paused. Getting out the words that I needed to say seemed so difficult that I might as well have had a tube stuck down my throat.

"Jenny," I said at last, "I don't know what happened to me at the conference today. But I'm sorry I let you down by not speaking up for what you wanted."

Just as they had when she had given me the note, her eyes began to tear.

"Jenny," I continued, "I'm not sure how you'll feel about this, especially given what's happened, but I'd like to say a prayer for you. I know that you've turned it down before. But honestly, at this point, I don't know what else to do."

Slowly, she pushed her hand across the sheet toward me. I felt relieved, knowing that she welcomed both my prayer and presence. I moved my hand forward in response, making sure not to place it on top of hers; she had little enough control of her environment as it was. But suddenly, as my fingers slid beneath her palm, her face contorted in a soundless howl. Her brittle bones unable to withstand even so slight a touch, she instantly jerked her hand away.

"Oh, my God, Jenny, I'm so sorry!" I exclaimed. Instead of reducing her suffering, I had only increased it, along with my own in the bargain. But for the fact she had responded positively to my offer only a moment before, I would have skipped the prayer entirely. Now, though, I was obliged, and I knew whatever prayer I said had to be truthful to what was happening. While I have seen the gravely-ill miraculously recover, the formulaic words of the *MiSheberach* requesting a speedy restoration to full health seemed wanting taken by themselves alone. Trying to think of something else, *something more*, to say, I sat silently for several minutes. Finally, the words of another prayer came into my mind. Those words rang truer not only to Jenny's condition but, more important, to her wishes:

"May the One who blessed our ancestors, Abraham and Sarah, Isaac and Rebecca, Jacob and Rachel and Leah, bless and heal Jenny, the daughter of Abraham and Sarah. May the Holy One, Blessed be He, guard and protect her and remove from her all her pain and suffering." I waited before continuing; of all the words I had spoken during my time with Jenny, the next ones would be hardest. "And when her soul departs, may it be with a kiss from Heaven. May the Compassionate One grant her peace when she departs this world and peace when she enters the next." Jenny nodded with what little strength she had. Her eyes teared once more.

The first thing after rounds next morning, I went to tell Beth about what had happened. I wanted to make sure that, given the charged situation between the hospital and Jenny's family, Beth was aware not only of my visit with Jenny, but in particular, of Jenny's reaction when I went to touch her hand. However, virtually before I could say anything at all, Beth broke in to give me her news, "I had another meeting with Lois this morning."

"And?" I asked, half hoping that Lois had finally seen the futility of keeping her mother intubated.

"She's still not willing to take her off the vent." I had a hunch about what was coming next. Although Beth may have been trained as a social worker, her formal job title was in fact "Discharge Planner."

"So, fine," Beth went on, "if Lois and Debbie want to keep their mom on the vent, we're not going to fight it. Risk Management agrees; it would just be too messy and too costly. But as I told Lois, if it doesn't look like their mom is eventually going to get off the vent and get better, then the ICU is not the appropriate place for her to be. Instead, she needs to be taken to an acute long-term facility where they focus on taking care of people on ventilators."

"What did Lois say when you told her that?" I asked, again hoping that that stark choice might itself have gotten Lois to agree to have the vent removed.

Beth just laughed and shook her head. "What do you expect somebody like Lois to say? She told me I'd be hearing from her lawyer! But that's the kind of thing people like Lois tell discharge planners all the time. Eventually, reality sets in. She'll crack—although in her case, it will probably mean sending her mother down the road to 'Vents-R-Us.'"

Within a few days, Lois proved Beth correct. Rather than opting to remove the breathing tube from her mother, Lois chose to remove her mother from the hospital. Thus was Jenny's fragile frame born by ambulance over twenty miles of potholed freeway to a ventilator facility—where she died before the week was out. However Jenny may have entered the next world, she did not, despite my prayer, depart this one in peace.

The world of the ICU had made such a departure all but impossible. With its lights always on and its machines constantly going off, the ICU is the casino from hell, where the dice are continually being rolled on high-stakes wagers of life and death. For those patients with a chance of recovery, the odds, however long, are undoubtedly worth taking. But for those like Jenny simply trying to die in peace, the house more often than not stacks the deck against them.

For the sake of all the other "Jennys," I knew I needed to move to a different setting, one that offered greater probabilities for peace in the face of impending death. Not long after Jenny's own departure, I myself left the ICU and entered hospice chaplaincy.

5

Nick's Scars

I WALKED INTO THE office of my hospice, Evergreen, one small part of a much larger HMO. I sat down at my desk, picked up the phone, and dialed into my voicemail to retrieve my messages. A voice that only another computer could (mis)take for human announced, "You have one new message. To hear your message, press 1."

I did, after which an unmistakably human voice began, "Michael, this is Barb. I've got a new patient for you."

As our hospice's "intake social worker," Barb made first contact with new patients placed on our service by their physicians. Many new patients and their family members experienced being placed on hospice as having had their doctors wash their hands of them and having thus been handed a death sentence. As a result, when Barb entered a home, instead of being welcomed as somebody offering resources ranging from medical to spiritual, she was frequently met with suspicion, if not outright hostility, as yet another huckster of betrayal, a shill for the greatest fraud of all: hope for extended life.

Barb's first task therefore was to lay down a foundation of trust with patients and their families. That often meant setting, as a cornerstone, some discussion of the key question many patients harbored in their hearts or, more frequently, voiced openly with their lips: "When will I die?" Patients typically already knew that, due to Medicare regulations, they wouldn't have been deemed appropriate for hospice unless at least two physicians had judged them likely to die within six months. Still, "within six months" could also mean within six weeks, or days, or hours. So, even as Barb acknowledged the severity of a patient's illness, she also affirmed a reality virtually every hospice worker has seen with his or her own eyes: patients can remain relatively healthy well past the six month mark while some, in fact, get well enough to go off hospice altogether. Barb straightaway began establishing trust with patients and their families by addressing, without sophistry or evasion, a fundamental truth of human life: *nobody* can predict with certainty when somebody else will die.

Barb's initial visit, however, also involved answering someone else's most basic question—*ours*, the hospice team's. We absolutely had to know, for the sake of the patient's welfare, whether his or her home was safe. And yet, within that question nested several others. First, did the home's physical layout pose additional burdens for a very ill patient who, as time progressed, would probably get much sicker? For instance, which room would accommodate a large hospital bed, when needed, and how far would that place the patient from a bathroom? If the bed, for example, would fit only in a front living room while the bathrooms were in the back or, even worse, on an upstairs floor, how would the patient manage, if at all, to get to them?

But Barb had still another, more critical home safety issue: were the patient's daily caregivers, whether family members or close friends, safe to be around? Could they be considered physically and emotionally strong enough to cope with the stresses of tending daily to a gravely-ill loved one? Could they be relied upon to give the patient the typical panoply of prescription drugs at the proper times? Or ought they to be regarded as so untrustworthy they might even steal the patient's powerful narcotics for themselves? (Unbelievable as it sounds, it happens.) All those first impressions in that first encounter among patient, family, and intake social worker therefore counted, if not for everything, then close to it.

"The new patient's name," Barb's message continued, "is Nick D'Agati. He's a seventy-two-year-old man with prostate cancer. He's a Roman Catholic. He's not active in the church, though, because for a long time before they were married, he and his second wife, Marie, lived together. Rightly or wrongly, the two of them feel embarrassed to go to church on the one hand and rejected by the church on the other. Anyway, Mr. D'Agati says he'd like to see a chaplain."

Neither the request nor circumstance struck me as unusual. Most hospice patients who ask to see a chaplain have no church affiliation. Had they, they generally would have already sought out spiritual support from their own clergy. So why, then, did many of our hospice patients ask me to visit them, especially if like this one, their prior experience with religion had been a bad one? Some, no doubt, feared death. Even those who thought they had years before sloughed off their religious upbringing, suddenly found themselves firmly in its grip once more as the end—and maybe even Perdition itself!—approached. Other patients, perhaps less anxious about dying, wanted only a soothing "pastoral presence" at their bedside. But whether afraid of death or not, most hospice patients I encountered wanted ultimately just one thing: to die in peace.

Dying in peace might sound synonymous with dying free from physical pain, and clearly, part of dying peacefully means dying without the body snarled in agony. Patients and families rightly fear pain, not merely as human beings, but as those who may have personally witnessed loved ones suffer needlessly in hospitals, where the treatment of pain can run the gamut from incompetence to indifference and back again. Hospice, by contrast, specializes in pain management. All hospice workers, chaplains included, upon visiting a patient must, by mandate, ask one question before any other: "On a scale of '1' to '10', where is your pain today?"; a response of "3" or higher requires immediate action to lower the pain. In my case, that meant phoning the central office to have a doctor raise the dosage of the patient's prescribed pain-killer—or to prescribe a new drug altogether. Thus, as I can attest from my own experience, and more important, as innumerable families can attest from theirs, the vast majority of hospice patients meet their deaths without physical pain escorting them.

Not dying in physical pain, however, is not the same as dying in peace. For a cluster of patients, relieving pain involves more than administering the right drugs. The physical pain these patients suffer often reflects a deeper psychic pain. That kind of pain cuts to their soul, slashing at their sense of who they are. Every hospice worker has probably encountered such patients, and almost all of us have done our best to assuage those patients' torment.

Even so, these soul-tormented patients comprise the heart of a hospice chaplain's practice. And "practice" here means exactly that, like "practicing piano" or "practicing law": working repeatedly on perfecting certain skills to achieve excellence. The singular practice of sitting daily with the dying helps develop a hospice chaplain's skills in discerning why a soul suffers and in alleviating that suffering. Just as a physician may need to see a patient with a baffling ailment several times to diagnose and treat it properly, a chaplain likewise may require numerous visits to identify and relieve a patient's mysterious spiritual dis-ease correctly. Sometimes, in speaking with spiritually-troubled patients and their families, I would describe my goal of helping sick family members die in peace as "bringing them in for a smooth landing." For obvious reasons, though, I never told them that, where the level of spiritual suffering is too high to overcome, no place exists for anything but a crash landing.

What kind of spiritual needs—and what kind of landing—might Nick D'Agati have? As Barb's voicemail had been silent on these issues, so also was his chart in the central office file. Its "H&P" provided only the standard "name, rank, and serial number" particulars. Mr. D'Agati had spent his working life as a longshoremen at the Port of Oakland. After his first wife died, he had married Marie, also a widow. Between the two of them, the ensuing family embraced not only their many biological children from their previous respective marriages, but also their assorted step-children via their remarriage, along with a dozen or so grandchildren and step-grandchildren besides. Mr. D'Agati had been diagnosed with prostate cancer while in his mid-60s, and now, seven or eight years later, this relatively slow-growing cancer had metastasized. Still, the chart said nothing about why he wanted to see me. To find that out, I had no recourse but to schedule a visit.

I called the D'Agati home, and an older woman's voice answered. "Hello?"

"Hello," I said, launching into my standard self-introduction, "I'm Michael, and I'm with Evergreen Hospice. With whom am I speaking, please?"

I intentionally did not identify myself as the hospice chaplain. Who knew who might be on the other end of the line and whether the patient wanted his medical condition shared with anybody else?

The woman's voice replied, "This is Marie D'Agati."

"Mrs. D'Agati," I began, "when you and your husband met with our social worker Barb yesterday, do you remember her saying that hospice could offer you spiritual support if you wanted it?" I still was not about to show all my cards. Patients sometimes have their own reasons for not letting even those closest to them know of their desire to see a chaplain, lest such a request invite unwelcome interest. Although a patient might be dying, his or her right to confidentiality and privacy nonetheless remains very much alive.

Marie was easy, though. "Yes! Nick and I could use some spiritual support right now. Are you the chaplain?"

"Yes, I am," I promptly answered. "I'd like to come by to meet Nick and you. Can I talk with him to see what would be a good time?"

"Nick's sleeping right now. But we're not going anywhere tomorrow. Could you stop by in the morning around ten?"

"Sure, I'll see you then." I said "Goodbye," hung up the phone, and wrote down the appointment in my notebook.

The D'Agatis' home was a five-minute drive from our office via surface streets, a blessing since, as the sole chaplain at Evergreen, my "service area" encompassed 125 square miles, and sometimes, covering only a few miles of California freeway felt like being forever trapped in one of Dante's inner rings of Hell. I pulled out of our parking lot, and a few minutes later, I arrived at the entrance to the D'Agatis' subdivision. It was not, however, the gated entranceway to some posh, lawn-manicured community. In California, where main roads can routinely extend unbroken for tens of miles, low stucco walls separating them from even the most modest neighborhoods provide residents some relief from the running eyesores of strip mall after strip mall and gas stations without end.

The tiny web of streets leading to the D'Agati home reflected the aspirations of the working class people living there as well as their pride in having realized those aspirations: cozy, well-maintained homes with equally well-kept yards and gardens. The houses also mirrored the individual tastes of their occupants. As I walked up the sidewalk to the D'Agatis' front door, a sudden, loud croak that sounded like it must have come from a giant mutant frog straight out of a 1950s horror movie nearly took my breath away. When I turned and looked down behind me, there was a frog all right: breadbox-sized and plastic.

"Oh, don't mind that," a warm, male voice said.

Looking up, I saw standing in front of me a stocky, powerfully-built man holding the screen door open. He had a head full of gunmetal gray hair, complemented by a sienna complexion. "The thing's a gift from my kids. It has a sensor or something in it, and every time somebody walks up the sidewalk to the house, it makes that sound."

"Mr. D'Agati?" I asked.

"Just call me Nick, Father."

Tickled, I replied, "First, I'm not a priest, and more important, if I get to call you Nick, then you ought to be able to call me Michael."

I walked inside the house, and it was every bit as warm and inviting as the man who lived there. Family pictures and keepsakes filled the living room, and from around the corner opening onto a homey kitchenette appeared a small, white-haired woman wearing oversized, blue-framed glasses.

"I'm Marie," she said, smiling at me. "Would you like to come into the kitchen for a cup of coffee?"

I was more than happy to accept, to feel so welcomed. It doesn't always happen that way.

No ubiquitous, automatic-drip coffee maker sat on the D'Agatis' kitchen counter. Instead, Marie went to a kitchen cabinet, took down a jar of "old-fashioned" freeze-dried crystals and three mugs. In each, she measured out a teaspoon before pouring boiling water from a nearby teakettle on the stove. We sat down around the kitchen table, sipping coffee as the D'Agatis made small talk.

Marie asked me, "Did you have trouble finding the place?"

Nick cut in, "Marie, the kids' frog startled Michael. We gotta' do something about that damn thing!"

Then it was my turn.

"Finding your place was easy, Marie. It's close to our office. And looking back on it, Nick, the frog's pretty funny. You know, on some days, I can use whatever humor I can find. So let me apologize for asking you a serious question now, but it's my first visit with you. As far as today goes, Nick, how would you rate your pain on the '1' to '10' scale, with '10' being the worst?"

Nick looked up, and his voice turned somber, "I guess I'm OK right now, but last night wasn't very good. Now don't get me wrong. Dr. Shapiro looks after me, and I really like him a lot. But ever since he put me on this new medication, I just have to pee all the time."

Dr. Shapiro, an oncologist, was our hospice medical director, a regulation-mandated position. While Dr. Shapiro technically bore ultimate responsibility for the medical care of all of Evergreen Hospice's patients, several had formerly been his own individual patients, and these he continued to see personally. A quiet, even shy man, Dr. Shapiro was a practicing Jew whose religious values helped shape the way he cared for patients. For instance, every Sabbath morning at his synagogue, he would have at least one of his patients, whether Jewish or not, mentioned by first name (so as to maintain confidentiality) in the special prayers for healing. Although Dr. Shapiro recognized these patients would probably die, he believed deeply in a God capable of healing, and more profoundly, he understood that healing and curing are not necessarily the same.

"Yeah, I like Dr. Shapiro, too," I said in agreement. "But it must be tough not being able to sleep at night."

"It makes it really hard on me during the day," Nick continued. "I'm a lot more tired, and it gets in the way of my daily routine."

"What's that?" I asked.

"I like to drive down to the 7-11 and buy a newspaper and a lotto ticket."

Amused, I asked with a grin, "Ever win anything?"

"Michael, that's not the point. The point is I *like* to do it. Sometimes when I'm out driving I see some guys in the neighborhood I know. They're gardening in front of their houses or just walking down the street, and I can go over and say 'Hello' to them."

"Oh, I see," I said, having been set straight. "What else do you like to do?"

Nick's eyes lit up. "I like to go to see the A's play," he said, referring to Oakland's baseball team. "I've been a fan for years. Always had season tickets. But now, it gets harder and harder for me to go. At first, I was un-comfortable because I couldn't pee. My ankles got so swollen. Then they gave me these new pills to take, and now I have to pee all the time. I've got a friend who has some seats, and he says I can use them any time I want. I have an idea where they're located, but I don't know how easy it would be to get to the john every time I'd need to. I guess I'm just waiting until I feel a little stronger to go out and take in a game. I really want to see the A's play the Yankees and beat those sons o' bitches."

And that was pretty much it for my first visit with Nick . . . and for several visits thereafter. Week after week, he and I would schedule a visit together, and week in, week out, we would talk—*he* would talk—about the A's and how their season was going. We might say a little prayer at the end of our visit, but that was about as far as things got "spiritually."

So why did Nick keep insisting on seeing me each week? As many women know from maddening experience with men, getting us to talk about our feelings can be more than just a little difficult. For many American men, a John Wayne-like stoicism exemplifies manhood par excellence. After all, except for throwing an occasional punch in righteous indignation, what other emotion did "the Duke" ever display? More to the point, can anyone even remotely imagine the Duke admitting he feared death (or anything else, for that matter), much less complaining—or Heaven forefend!—crying about it? For a man of Nick's background and generation, a man who had been both stevedore and paterfamilias, the very prospect of having to talk about his feelings ironically might have brought on the most terrifying feeling of all.

No one, though, should jump to the simplistic conclusion that Nick kept calling on me because if and when he ever were to "share" his feelings, he would do so only with another man. Nick plainly had plenty of other men around him in whom he could confide, from his grown sons and grandsons to his old buddies from the docks. So why me? While my being a man may have been part of Nick's continuing desire to see me, my being in his eyes "a man of the cloth" played, as things turned out, a far greater part.

Over the course of our visits, I had the growing sense that something was weighing heavily on Nick, something that from his perspective, only I—or someone like me—could help lift off him and thus help him die in peace. Invariably, every time I visited, his conversation veered toward baseball, that game American males have traditionally, for generations, taught their sons to play, almost as a rite of passage. But whenever I tried to steer our talk to Nick's taking in an A's' game, he always changed the subject. I knew that Nick had raised the frequent urination issue with his female nurse; following each visit, she, like all the team's members, left messages for everybody else, as required by regulation. I knew, moreover, that Nick would never talk about his urinary frequency problems with a female chaplain, because, as he once somewhat bashfully told me, "Chaplains are about, you know, the 'spiritual' and not the 'physical' side of things." For all that, however, the mystery remained of what so oppressed Nick's spirit—and what he wanted me to do to remove it.

And then one week, I drove up to his house, looked at the *Oakland Tribune* sports section to check how the A's were doing in the standings, got out of the car, walked up the sidewalk past the croaking frog, knocked on the screen door, and waited for several minutes for someone to come open it. Had Marie been home, she would have answered. While I knew she loved Nick and took good care of him despite her own age and maladies, she had, over the course of my last few visits, made herself scarce, as though sensing Nick needed to be alone with me to talk.

Finally, Nick appeared. He was walking very slowly, his face drooping down, indeed his whole body stooped over, looking as though gravity itself were pulling him inexorably toward the ground.

"Hello, Michael," he mumbled. "I'm not doing very well at all. Why don't you come in, and we'll talk."

After we had taken our usual places at the kitchen table, I asked, "What's wrong? Are you in pain?"

With a long, weary sigh, he responded, "Nothing physical. Just other stuff."

"Like what?"

"I can't get around any more like I used to," he said. "Forget about going down to get the lotto ticket. The only place I can get to is the toilet. And then, I just tire out right away."

Then he told a story about what truly troubled him far more revealing than anything having to do with urinary problems.

"The kids," he said, "are upsetting me a lot right now. They're arguing over who gets a ring I have. I want to give it to one of my grandsons. He's a real good boy. But some of my children, along with Marie's, think that the ring should go to one of them instead. In the old days, I would just have told them, 'That's the way it's going to be whether you like it or not!' Now I just don't have the strength to do it, and it really hurts me."

While Nick could accept his death, he could not accept what the dying process might mean for him. When he had worked the docks as foreman supervising others, who had ever told *him* what to do? When he had been clan chieftain with other family members in his charge, who had ever directed, much less challenged, *him*?

The temptation to offer a bromide at such moments can be overwhelming: "Oh, Nick, don't talk like that! You're still the same head of the family you've always been, and your children still love and respect you the way they always have." Though such a statement may give its speaker some relief, it hardly ever gives the sufferer any. She or he is probably in no mood to welcome it, let alone hear or heed it. Besides, what if, for instance, some of Nick's or Marie's children had never had much respect or love for the old man in the first place? Now, he could possibly be even more vulnerable to their hostility.

Resisting the desire "to say something comforting" means holding fast onto the patience required to sit in silence, waiting, listening for what might come next. A hospice chaplain must master the skill to hear another's heart speak its depth, for from its depths, the heart does not speak easily or often.

So after nodding to acknowledge that I had heard what Nick had said, I sat silently and waited for what more, if anything, might come. But as I saw the minutes sweeping by on the kitchen wall clock behind him, I concluded that Nick's disclosure about the family's wrangling over his ring had squeezed as much out of him as he could endure that day. Anyway, I had to negotiate fifteen miles of freeway to arrive even remotely on time for my next patient.

But then, as I was about to get up, Nick spoke up. He had something more to say, something even more tightly tethered to his sense of who he was than what he had just now revealed.

"You know, Michael," he began, "I don't blame my prostate cancer on anybody else but me. I should have had those tests, but I just didn't, and now I got cancer. But that's not the hardest part."

Nick halted, and drew a deep breath before continuing. "When I first got the word, the doctor who told me pointed down here." Again Nick stopped. He gestured toward his genitals. "Then the doctor just up and said to me, 'You don't need those two damn things anyway. We might as well cut them off.'"

Nick's voice grew fainter. "I'll tell you something, Michael. That happened eight years ago, and it still hurts me to think about it. Do you think it was right for that doctor to tell me that way?"

Silence again. But this time, the silence came from me. What could I say in the face of such an unspeakably heartless pronouncement whose soul-piercing wound Nick still felt almost a decade later? Finally, I said, "I'm sorry, Nick."

My response might seem banal, akin to asking someone "How are you?" when no concern genuinely exists regarding that person's welfare. But when I said to Nick, "I'm sorry," I offered those words not as some "throwaway line," and certainly not as an apology for anything I myself had done, nor even as an expression of regret for my HMO's having employed that bastard of a surgeon. No, when I spoke the words, "I'm sorry," I uttered them with their original meaning in mind: "It makes my heart sore."

For that is exactly what Nick's story had done to my heart. For eight years, he had been carrying the scar of the doctor's words as well as their surgical aftermath. Nick had been twice cut as a man.

Once more, Nick and I sat in silence. Neither of us had anything more to say; indeed, neither of us *could* say anything more that day.

During the visits that followed, the time spent in silence far exceeded the time spent in conversation. More precisely, Nick remained largely silent. Following his disclosure about his castration and the traumatic event leading up to it, his spiritual suffering, having been brought to the surface, seemed only to intensify, like a laceration of the skin that for the moment, at least, cannot bear to be touched or dressed, however tenderly, to help treat and relieve the pain. So Nick's spiritual wound lay exposed and raw, festering and infected further by depression.

I have seen many hospice patients beset by severe depression; and given their situations, why not? But I have also seen almost as many patients re-emerge with spirits raised—provided they have received the right support. Some of that support comes from the pharmacological expertise and experience that hospice physicians, nurses and apothecaries bring to patients in their care. Yet medication alone cannot supply all the support depressed patients need. Some support must come from other human beings, especially those closest to these patients. In other words, the timely spiritual interventions of family and friends may prove crucial in helping a loved one safely navigate through depression's straits.

Baseball was the one sure thing I knew, his depression notwithstanding, that still managed to buoy Nick's spirits, if only just a bit. As depleted as he was emotionally, an A's' win usually gave him the kind of renewed, albeit temporary, vitality a blood transfusion gives a leukemia patient. Nick sometimes spoke wistfully of his friend with the ballpark seats who had continued to invite him to come use them. But Nick's depression, coupled with his ongoing self-consciousness about his frequent need to urinate, provided a handy excuse for declining every invitation. Left to his own devices, Nick would, I feared, never make it out of his house to the ballpark—or anywhere else—but simply stay at home depressed, waiting for death to come get him.

So I began to wonder what steps might be needed to get Nick to a game. Before anything else, of course, he had to start taking the antidepressants Dr. Shapiro had recommended for him. But even assuming the drugs would work, I could foresee other challenges ahead: suppose Nick did somehow make it out to the stadium, how would he get to his friend's seats located in the upper deck? Next, how would he get each of his multiple medications taken at its proper time? And finally, how would he get to a toilet with ease during the many times he would likely have to use it?

But before I ever got the chance to address any of those issues fully and help Nick get on track for an A's' game—and maybe leave depression's province—everything got derailed by an unexpected roadblock: Vera, Nick's daughter. While Nick himself had agreed to start taking the anti-depressants, getting Vera to agree to let him take them was quite another matter. A large, domineering woman, Vera herself had had a bad reaction to anti-depressants some years before, and consequently, as she emphatically—and menacingly—told Nick's hospice nurse, "I'm sure as hell not going to stand around and let my sick father go through the same goddamn thing I did."

Hospice workers encounter many families with a Vera in them, someone who has assumed—or who has been assigned—the role of tenacious advocate for the patient's welfare. In fact, something would be wrong with a family were nobody to play that role. Families of the dying encounter some of the worst moments and choices any family can ever face. They are struggling against outsized odds in a bout they know they probably will lose. But Vera had acted so combatively toward her father's nurse as well as toward several other members of the hospice team that, as a last resort, the team asked me to try to gain her blessing with regard to the anti-depressants, because I, at least, came with a clean slate, having had no prior interactions with her, whether for good or ill.

Accordingly, I scheduled my next visit to the D'Agatis' home when I thought Vera might be present, which it turned out she was. Marie was present this time, too, along, of course, with Nick himself. Again today, Vera played the role of advocate. Whether the family had given her that role, or merely acquiesced, I could not tell. Nevertheless, once the preliminary introductions had been made, I began by intentionally speaking to Nick, hoping to focus the conversation primarily on his needs rather than on Vera's.

"So Nick," I began as always, "what's going on with you today?"

Vera would have none of it. "Well, why don't you just take a look at him. He's doing terrible."

Trying to acknowledge Vera's remark, while still trying to afford Nick an opportunity to speak for himself, I turned again to him and asked, "Nick, are you in pain?"

"No!" barked Vera. "But can't you see how down he is!"

For a chaplain, one of the hardest and yet easiest things to do at such a time is to take someone's anger without taking it personally. You are, after all, a convenient target. Clergy are expected to "be nice" and, whether they are Christian or not, "to turn the other cheek." More significant, many patients and families, whether theists or not, are angry with God in such circumstances, and because they may consciously or unconsciously perceive the chaplain as God's "stand-in," target him or her as the focus for their rage. Sometimes, I wished their rage over a loved one's impending death could have been directed justifiably toward me, because then presumably, I really would have had the power to take the steps necessary to prevent it. But no more than Vera did I possess the ability to stop Nick from dying, and certainly, no less than she did I want him to keep on living.

Keeping my voice calm and even, I turned back to Vera and affirmed what she had said. "I know your dad is depressed. He and I have talked about that over the last two or three times I've visited him. And it's clearly normal for someone in this situation to become depressed, but it's also normal for them to come out of it—*if* they can get the right kind of support from family and medication."

"You mean drugs?" Vera retorted. "I told somebody else in your hospice—I don't remember who—I'm not about to let my father go near those anti-depressants. Some goddamn doctor had me on them, and they messed me up for a long time."

"Obviously, I can't speak about your experience," I replied. "But I do know that everybody's biochemistry is different, and that there are lots of different anti-depressants out there. And you know what? We're not talking about your dad taking these drugs for a long time, but just long enough to help pull him up out of the funk he's fallen into now. As I understand it—and I admit, I'm not a member of the medical staff—these drugs generally take effect within two weeks or so. So why not at least give your dad the chance to feel a little better so he can do something we all think would be good for him—you know, like go to an A's' game? What do you think?"

To my relief, Vera agreed. "Well, I guess for a short amount of time it wouldn't be too bad."

"Good," I continued. "If you give me a phone, I'll contact our office right now, and let them call in a prescription to our pharmacy so the medicine can be delivered out here by this afternoon. Meanwhile, why don't *you* start working on getting in touch with your father's friend to reserve your dad and you some tickets for a game within the next few weeks?"

Having thus gotten Vera to concur with Nick's taking the anti-depressants, I knew I also had to give her a "task." I had a hunch that a revised version of the old adage might best fit her: "Like father, like daughter." I would have bet that she, too, like her father in his heyday, had a foreman's attitude. If a job needed doing, *she* would oversee it and take responsibility for its being done right. Without my assigning her the project of arranging the logistics for the game, I feared she would go back to her previous job of barring her father from taking the anti-depressants. As I led our customary group prayer before leaving, I offered a silent one of my own that our pharmacy would deliver the anti-depressants on time that afternoon so that Nick could start taking them before Vera had a change of heart.

Thank God—and the pharmacy driver—the anti-depressants did arrive as scheduled, Nick did start to take them immediately, and best of all, he did begin to feel their effects within a matter of days. Meanwhile, Vera, bless her, made all the necessary arrangements for the game. And who better for the home team to play than the hated Yanks—whom the A's slaughtered, much to the joy of one and all.

During the summer of 1961, when I was eleven, I never ventured far from a TV or transistor radio so that I could follow the fortunes of my beloved Cincinnati Reds, who were on their way to their first National League pennant in over twenty years. On days when the Reds won their games during that baseball season, my spirits went way up; on days when they lost, I would go far down into the dumps. Some hospice patients respond to their illnesses that way, soaring on emotional updrafts on days they feel better, free-falling in despair on days they don't. I often told my patients they would be best served by trying to respond to their sickness in a more steady, constant way, enjoying a good day as it came, suffering through a bad one for what it was and nothing more. But that kind of even, balanced coping is particularly difficult for the terminally ill because they know that, in the end, a complete season, let alone a winning one, is probably beyond their grasp.

Certainly Nick knew that. Although he enjoyed the trip out to the ballpark immensely and felt good for a week or so afterwards, he realized that his present high spirits would no more persist than would his current relatively high level of physical strength. True enough, within a couple weeks following the game, Nick's mood grew, if not more depressed, definitely more subdued as his mobility became ever more circumscribed. He could no longer drive not only to get his lotto ticket but even to see his friends. He could no longer exit or re-enter his home without using a wheelchair ramp his grandson had built for him. He couldn't even get around inside his own house without the aid of a walker.

And yet, the trip to the baseball game had managed to accomplish one thing. It re-kindled in Nick an ember of his sense of maleness, of manliness, which vigorously re-asserted itself in a particular field of action that Nick now staked out as his and his alone: making the arrangements for his funeral. As if reaffirming himself as head-of-household, Nick resolved to spare Marie both the hardship of having to make the arrangements herself and the potentially hard work of keeping their often contentious brood at bay should their children try to fight out the details of his burial following his death.

Nick displayed what I suspected had been his lifelong sense of what it meant to be "a man" in yet another way. It showed itself in his perseverance to be buried as a Catholic. Although he believed that his "unsanctioned" relationship with Marie prior to their marriage, combined with the fact that they hadn't been actively involved with any church for years, might make it difficult to find a priest to conduct the service, none of that deterred him. Remaining tough-minded despite several initial refusals, he still eventually got hold of a priest to officiate. An acquaintance, as it turned out, worked at a local cemetery, where he, in turn, knew a priest who in due course agreed to preside at a memorial service in the cemetery's chapel.

I therefore considered everything in place for bringing Nick in for one of those smooth landings. I thought we had broken through the clouds, gently descending now with the runway lights ahead in sight, guiding us safely home. It was straightforward. It was routine. I had done it so many times before. I could almost feel the wheels touching down.

Then suddenly, a violent windshear hit . . . and it hit not Nick, but *me*.

In the midst of one of our by-now customary conversations—"The A's are doing pretty good the last few days"; "The kids are behaving themselves OK"; "The priest is all lined up"—Nick's voice unexpectedly dropped as his face filled with chagrin. "God, Michael, I just hate having to pee all the time."

"Why? What do you mean?" I asked. "Is it the nuisance of it? Or is it painful? Or is it something else?"

He pointed to his groin. "I just can't stand looking at the goddamn cut-up ugly thing."

I didn't know what to say. But I didn't have to, because Nick knew exactly what *he* wanted to say. "I want to show you just how bad it looks."

Nothing could have prepared me for those words. Had I known beforehand Nick was going to speak them, I honestly don't think I could have made the visit. As it was, I just wanted to run out of the house. But I didn't, not out of any sense of "professionalism," nor even out of any feeling of "compassion," but because I simply froze. Of course, had I turned and run away, I would have merely confirmed Nick's self-perception that his prior surgery and his ever-worsening disease had so disfigured him that he was indeed too hideous to look at.

Nick removed his trousers, then the diaper he was wearing for incontinence. Aghast and yet somehow mesmerized, I gazed at his purpled, bloated penis. In his own eyes, and now in mine, too, his castration eight years earlier ("You don't need those two damn things anyway!") had neutered him. Now, his increasingly frequent need to urinate relentlessly reminded him of that every time he pulled down his pants. Nick's compulsion to show me his physical scar scored into his skin reflected his need to expose me to the other scar gashed into his spirit. For a man like Nick, the pain from that spiritual scarring was far worse than any physical suffering attributable to his cancer.

But not just for a man like Nick. For a man like me, too. In the past, I had visited women who had had mastectomies. They had told me how, as a result of such procedures, they no longer saw themselves as women. Naturally, I listened attentively and empathetically. Clearly, though, I am not a woman, I do not have breasts like theirs, and I will never experience the significance of a mastectomy the way they had. So while I could empathize with these female patients "as human beings," I could in no way wholly grasp the anguish they carried with them.

I do, however, have a penis. When I saw Nick's mutilated penis, I needed no vicarious act of empathy to "understand" his suffering. I felt it with an immediacy that shot through my gut and soul. And it hurt. It hurt so much, in fact, that I began to cry, for Nick *and* for myself. Then Nick started sobbing, too. For the next several minutes, all we did was sit there weeping, and as we sat there, we embraced each other tightly. Finally, we let go of each other, sitting in the silence of agony's relief. As usual, our visit ended with a prayer, only this time spoken barely at the level of a whisper, as if all that had needed to be expressed more loudly had already had its say.

The next time I came to see Nick, I approached with some apprehension. Would there be something else he would share that would hit so close to home? With each step I took toward the front door, I felt my stomach tighten, and when, just as I was about to ring the bell, the plastic frog croaked, I felt almost as startled by it as I had the first time I visited the D'Agati home.

But Nick came to the door relatively quickly, with no sign of the distress I had seen before. On the contrary, as we talked, I got a sense of what his old, healthy self might have been like. He had taken complete charge of making all the final preparations for his funeral, from purchasing the burial plot to picking the music and readings for the service to tying up the loose ends of engaging the cemetery's "on-call" Catholic priest to officiate. But perhaps most important, not only for the arrangements once he died but also for himself while he still lived, he had told everyone in his family in no uncertain terms, "*That's* how it's going to be!"—including *which* grandson would get his ring.

I replied with all my heart, "I'm really glad to hear it, Nick. I know that when you die, what you have done now will make things easier for your family, especially for Marie. Since she won't have to focus on making any funeral arrangements once you're gone, she'll be able to attend to the job she'll need to do then most—I mean, mourn the loss of somebody she loved most. How could you possibly better show your love for her, or for your children, for that matter?"

Nick sighed, "Thanks, Michael." Then he paused, stared at me, and said, "And now I've got a favor to ask of you."

"Ask away," I answered. "If I can, I'll do it."

Because Nick meant so much to me, I absolutely wanted to help him if I could. But how? After all, he had just finished telling me that he had made all the arrangements for his funeral, and as far as I could determine, whatever spiritual wounds had previously pained him had been salved, at least for now. Consequently, as on so many other occasions, all I could do was sit and wait and listen.

Nick waited a while before finally speaking. "You know, I guess there are going to be some people getting up to say some things about me, eulogies or whatever you call them. Hell, you can't keep people like Vera from talking! And I suppose some of my other kids and some of my buddies might want to say something, too."

"So," I thought to myself, "Nick wants me to give a eulogy. Sure, I've done that lots of times before. No problem."

But that's not what Nick wanted at all.

"Michael," he said, "I'm not asking you to stand up and give some damn speech. There will be enough of that as it is. Instead, would you do this for me? Would you just get up and say I was a good guy?"

This longshoremen, this "tough guy," had done it to me again: he had brought me to the point of tears.

"Nick," I answered, "if I'm able to attend the funeral—if I'm not with someone else or someplace else—I couldn't feel more privileged than to have the chance to say that, because you know something? Only a good guy would care that that's all that would be said about him. And to me, that's exactly what you are."

We both smiled. Although both of us may well have smiled simultaneously during some previous visit, the only instance I can remember with certainty was that one.

I saw Nick three or four more times after that. I left Evergreen to take another job. Nick died a few months later.

He was a good guy.

6

Lucille's Teeth

"IT'S THE MAN FROM hostage!" Lucille cried out to no one in particular as she saw me come into the activities room of the Pleasant Valley Nursing Home. She did not have dementia. Instead, she had a sense of humor. In a nursing home, distinguishing between the two is sometimes not so easy.

Once, I went to make an initial visit to an elderly woman in a different facility. Before entering her room, I knocked on its doorframe, introduced myself, and asked if I might come in to speak with her. She nodded "Yes." And yet, despite my best efforts to strike up a conversation, for the next fifteen minutes she simply sat on the edge of her bed, stock-still. As a last resort, I asked her if she would like me to say a prayer for her. "I say my own prayers!" she snapped. "That's good." I replied. Then, attempting to elicit a few more words from her, I inquired, "What prayers do you say?" "Our Father, who art in Heaven," she began reciting, "hallowed be thy name—" She halted as though fumbling for what followed next. After a few seconds, she started up again: "Our Father, who art in Heaven, hallowed be . . ." Once more, she faltered. I made a suggestion: "Why don't we try saying it together?" She shook her head in agreement, and the two of us began in unison: "Our Father, who art in Heaven, hallowed be thy name, thy kingdom come, thy will be done . . ." Midway through, I ceased speaking while the woman continued without misstep to the prayer's conclusion. Now that she was talking, I wanted to try and keep her chatting. "Is there anything else you'd like to talk about?" "I want . . . ," she said and then trailed off into what sounded like gibberish to me. "I'm sorry," I replied, "I didn't get that. Would you please repeat it for me?" Again, she said, "I want . . . ," and again her words dissolved into gobbledygook. Once more, I apologized for not being able to comprehend her. "Would you like me to get someone, a nurse or aide perhaps, who might understand you better?" She looked straight into my eyes and said with frustration, "Go fuck yourself." For the "resident" of a nursing home, madness may furnish the sanest coping device of all.

Approximately eleven million Americans reside in nursing homes for some period of their lives, especially at or near the end of their lives.[1] By 2020, that number may explode as some fifty-three million "baby boomers" turn sixty-five,[2] with perhaps ninety per cent of them experiencing slow declines, punctuated by periodic crises, before eventually dying from such illnesses as heart disease or emphysema.[3] During the course of their protracted deterioration, their families, unable—or unwilling—to care for them in their own homes, may choose to have them transferred to nursing homes instead. The elderly may reluctantly agree, not wishing to become "a burden" to their children, an idea more horrifying to many Americans than the thought of death itself.

Thus, numerous hospice patients end up as residents of nursing homes. Of these, dementia patients comprise a large number, but a growing segment falls within the catch-all diagnosis of "failure to thrive"— patients whose bodies, simply put, are just plain giving out, no matter the measures taken to sustain them. So it was with the eighty-eight-year-old body of Lucille Larkin.[4]

Lucille was a resident of the Pleasant Valley Nursing Home, located on a wide street off a major thoroughfare in San Francisco's East Bay.

1. While no definitive figures exist, see, e.g., Michael Kinsley, "Mine is Longer than Yours," *The New Yorker*, April 7, 2008, 38–43. As Kinsley writes (42), "It starts with so-called 'independent living,' and runs through 'assisted living' to the nursing home, with possible detours through 'home health care' and 'rehab,' and thence to the hospital and points beyond." Kinsley knows better than most the topography of the area: he has Parkinson's disease.

2. See Dr. Jerald Winakur of The Center for Medical Humanities and Ethics at the University of Texas Health Science Center, "What Are We Going to Do with Dad?: No Pat Answers for the 'Old Old'," *The Washington Post*, Sunday, 7 August 2005, B01: "As we baby boomers go about our lives, frozen into our routines of work and family responsibilities, a vast inland sea of elders is building. By 2020 there will be an estimated 53 million Americans older than 65, 6.5 million of whom will be 'old old [i.e., older than eighty-five].' . . . America will be inundated with old folks, each with a unique set of circumstances, medical and financial."

3. Cf. statistics compiled by Vitas, one of the largest providers of hospice care in the U.S.

4. "Lucille" is unique among the patients in this book, reflecting no single individual, but instead a composite of various nursing home residents I have met in dozens of different SNFs. In other words, what happens in the following account to this "Lucille" happened in one way or another to other "Lucilles" elsewhere.

Pleasant Valley had a smallish, but well-tended lawn with two strategi-cally-planted shade trees standing opposite one another, their branches overarching the sidewalk leading up to the facility's main entrance. As a nursing home, Pleasant Valley comes under the formal rubric used by professional healthcare providers: "Skilled Nursing Facility." But in the everyday lingo of professionals, a place like Pleasant Valley goes by the acronym, "SNF," which is pronounced exactly the way it looks—"*sniff*"— ironically providing a handy means of initially gauging the quality of care of such an institution. Hence, as I entered Pleasant Valley's cramped lobby, I took a whiff of the air around me and detected no stink of urine, indicat-ing residents left to sit or lie in their own waste, nor stench of ammonia, signifying efforts to dilute urine's odor. But as I scanned Pleasant Valley's reception area, I saw over a dozen of its wheelchair-bound residents ar-rayed randomly around its main nurses' station, signaling perhaps too-few staff to properly monitor the nonambulatory or mentally-impaired residents in its care. My first impression, therefore, of Pleasant Valley? It struck me as neither exceptionally good nor bad, but as just another SNF.

Before visiting Lucille for the first time, I wanted to look at her chart to learn something about her history, both personal and physical. But the nursing station was not a library reading room. Jammed with dozens of thick charts representing residents who had lived at the SNF for years, the close quarters of the station left precious little space for chart review— space made more meager still by the battery of wheelchairs packed tightly round it. And yet, far greater than those physical barriers to my reviewing Lucille's chart lay an institutional one potentially more daunting: get-ting the attention *and* assistance of the Pleasant Valley staff. Notoriously comprised of overworked, underpaid aides augmented by a handful of harried nurses, SNF staff frequently register indifference to requests of residents and non-residents alike. But as I wedged my way between two wheelchairs up to the desk, a nurse standing behind the counter spotted me and called out, "Hello, Doctor! Who are you here to see today?"

As a (white) male in the disproportionately female-staffed world of nursing homes,[5] I was frequently mistaken for a physician, shown def-erence, and, contrary to regulations protecting residents' confidentiality, given unimpeded access to their charts. Lifting up the hospice ID badge

5. —and hospices.

hanging from the cord around my neck, I answered, "Thank you, but I'm not a physician. I'm a chaplain with Wellspring Hospice, and I'm here to visit one of your residents, Ms. Louise Larkin. Might I please see her chart?"

I had chosen my words to the SNF nurse carefully in referring to Lucille as one of "your residents" rather than as one of "our patients." At some SNFs, staff show less attentiveness to the needs of residents once they are placed on hospice, assuming, consciously or not—but in any case wrongly—that care for those residents now falls entirely to hospice. I had another reason for choosing my words to the nurse quite cautiously. My *requesting* to see Lucille's chart went beyond common courtesy. From the beginning, I wanted to do everything I could to lower the prospects of any potential SNF-hospice turf war in which Lucille might become "collateral damage."

Now that the nurse knew she was addressing a chaplain rather than a doctor, she dispensed with any further niceties. Mutely, she turned around, lifted Lucille's chart from the shelf behind the desk, and unceremoniously plopped it down on the countertop between us. The chart, clad in a dark green, three-ring binder, must have been three inches thick. But our hospice's portion constituted only a few slim pages of it, because Lucille had come on to our census a mere couple days before. While I had neither the time—nor space—to lay open the chart and read it from cover to cover, I took what limited opportunity I had to skim its most recent entries, along with Lucille's "H&P," i.e., her medical history and physical examination on admission to the SNF. A resident of Pleasant Valley for the past three years, Lucille had originally been admitted after having fallen repeatedly due to an underlying chronic condition—the fragility associated with old age.[6] A week ago, two physicians had deemed her "hospice appropriate," diagnosing her as likely terminal within the next six months. And yet, patients with a terminal diagnosis of "failure to thrive" may often live far beyond the original prognosis. Consequently, in initial increments of ninety and then later sixty days, Medicare typically extends such patients' hospice benefit. But who could say what benefit Lucille might receive from Pleasant Valley's care as she died there slowly over the months that lay ahead?

6. See Muriel R. Gillick, *Lifelines: Living Longer, Growing Frail, Taking Heart* (New York: Norton, 2000).

Lucille's Teeth

The nurse's voice interrupted my reading of the chart: "She's in Room 42, Bed B." It was the signal to move on. I signed the visitors' log and tucked Lucille's binder on the ledge beneath the countertop where, following my visit, I could easily retrieve it to chart my progress note before I left.

I walked down a tapioca-colored corridor that branched out into three more hallways. Each looked the same: narrow, low-ceilinged, windowless, devoid of any light save for that emanating from fluorescent tubes hanging overhead. As I made a series of false starts looking for Lucille's room, I heard no speech or talk of any kind, but only an occasional shriek, coming perhaps from a dementia patient inside the grotto of residents' rooms that pocketed the passageways. Chancing at last on a SNF aide with the lunchtime meal cart, I asked directions to Room 42, Bed B.

"Oh, Doctor [Again!] you mean Lucille's room! Straight down the hall, last room on your left, the bed by the door."

I followed the aide's instructions to the room, coming finally to my destination. Before entering, I knocked to announce myself and request permission to come in—exactly as I would have done had Lucille lived under her own roof instead of Pleasant Valley's. I raised my voice to make myself heard through the room's half-closed, heavy wooden door. "Ms. Larkin," I said, "My name is Michael Goldberg, and I'm a chaplain with Wellspring Hospice. May I come in?"

From inside, a lively voice responded, "Yes, that's fine. Come have a seat!"

Poking my head around the door, I saw lying in the bed before me a woman whose eyes matched her voice. Gay and energetic, they seemed to belie not only her wispy white hair, her reed-like arms, and the canals of creases that crisscrossed her face, but her very age itself.

"Thank you, Ma'am," I replied, "I'm pleased to have the chance to meet you. Our intake social worker, Carol, said you wanted to see me."

"Oh, yes! I'm glad to have the company!"

As I stepped all the way inside the room, I saw it was, in reality, only half a room, the whole having been bisected by a hospital curtain, from whose other side I could hear a low, intermittent moan. Lucille's side was barely large enough for her bed, a nightstand, and a chair, along with a bathroom shared with her "roommate" beyond the curtain.

As I pulled up the chair to sit down beside her bed and begin our talk, Lucille stopped me. "Wait a second! I need to put my choppers in!"

She turned away, reached into the nightstand, snatched out a pair of dentures and, only after having fitted them into her mouth securely, faced my way again. "How do you like my new teeth?" she asked, smiling warmly, even slightly coyly. "I got them yesterday. I know it's silly to be vain at my age, but they make me feel better."

"What's wrong with that? They look terrific!" I answered her in all honesty. "But, tell me, what can *I* do to help make you feel better? As I said, my colleague, Carol, mentioned that you wanted to see a chaplain."

"And as *I* said," she rejoined, "I'm glad to have the company—*any* company. Even after having lived here for so many years, I still haven't gotten used to feeling more or less alone. And since I got put on hospice, I feel more isolated than ever. The other residents tend to steer clear of me. They already think about illness, death, and loss enough as it is. Why should they invest in a relationship with somebody who's terminal? And who knows? Maybe the nurses and aides think about me the same way, too. Or maybe, they figure that from here on in, the hospice staff will take care of me."

I noticed a photograph in a tarnished silver frame on the nightstand. As I glanced around the room, it was the sole picture or personal effect I saw. How could she not help but feel alone?

"Who's this in the photo?" I asked her gently.

"It's my family—my husband, Jack, who died thirty years ago, and my two boys, Phil, who's in Arizona, and his older brother, Brian, who's back on the East Coast in New York. I don't get to see them much. Apart from the distance, they have families of their own and lead very busy lives."

"How do they feel about your being on hospice?"

"They're concerned, of course, but what can they do? We talk by phone about once a week."

"Do you have any friends in the area who come by to see you?"

"Not really. I've outlived them all."

I tried to think of people in addition to myself who might provide Lucille with increased companionship.

"Besides continuing my own visits to you, I can request a hospice volunteer to drop by and keep you company. Would you like that?"

The trace of a denture-filled smile crossed her face. "That might work. I guess it depends on whether or not the volunteer and I hit things off!"

"Of course. Like everything else with hospice, it's totally your call." I made a mental note to contact Twyla, our hospice's Volunteer Coordinator, to request someone come by and "audition" for Lucille.

I thought of another resource that might provide her with companionship and, even perhaps, some comfort.

"Before you moved here, did you belong to a church whose clergy I might call to come visit you?"

"For about twenty years, I went to Faith United Fellowship. You might have driven past it—it's less than five minutes away. But I haven't belonged for years. After all this time, I don't feel comfortable about having you contact the pastor or anybody else at the church."

"As I said, Ms. Larkin, it's totally your call. But are you OK with my coming back to spend time with you?"

"So far, everything seems copasetic. Go ahead and put me on your dance card. And stop calling me 'Ms. Larkin'—call me 'Lucille', the same as everybody else does."

"It's a deal," I promised. "And from now on, you'll be one of my regulars."

"Okay, then, Michael, if I may call you that," she continued, without awaiting my reply, "I'm honestly not afraid of death. I've heard the staff here joke that people who die in a nursing home never go to hell— they've already been there! And *that's* what really scares me. I can't bear the thought of being here practically all alone until I die."

Trying to reassure her, I reiterated my commitment to visit her frequently as well as to seek a hospice volunteer who would also stop by often. In passing, I said that should she change her mind, I would be glad to call her former church and inquire whether its clergy or members could drop in to give her some more companionship.

"Thank you, but I can't have you do that," Lucille said as though embarrassed. "I belonged to the church only because of the opportunities it had for socializing—the Ladies' Club, the pot-lucks, and the like. In fact, I don't think I ever went to any worship services there. And as long as we're at it, I *really* appreciate your not going all 'Holy Joe' and offering to pray with me. I'm genuinely grateful for the time you've spent with me, but, speaking truthfully, I'm feeling a little tuckered out, and I'd like to get some rest."

"That's fine, Lucille. I'll be back next week." Whether out of the comfort provided by that knowledge or from the satisfaction given by the new dentures, she smiled once more before I left.

I said good-bye and retraced my steps back to the nurses' station out front. Reaching for the ledge under the countertop, I lifted up Lucille's binder from the spot where I had left it and made a brief entry in my hospice's as-yet small section. Then, I turned back to the thick binder's very first page, tore off a piece of scratch paper from a nearby pad, and copied the contact phone numbers for Lucille's sons, recorded upon her admittance three years prior. After I finally caught the attention of a nurse, I handed her the binder to replace to its proper alphabetical slot among all the other charts shelved on the drab green metal case behind her. Thanking her, I logged out, squeezed through the wheelchairs of the dozing and deranged, and headed toward the parking lot.

Once inside my car, I took out my cell phone to call Brian as well as Phil. I didn't want to phone them from inside the SNF, because its confines afforded me no haven within which to collect my thoughts or to protect Lucille's privacy. In the end, my location didn't matter; I wound up reaching neither brother. Instead, I left on each one's voicemail a message broadly outlining my visit. In addition, I left each one my phone number with an invitation to call me back for more details. In the ensuing week, I never heard from either of the two.

As a result, when I returned to see Lucille for our next visit, I knew nothing more about her than I had at the end of our first meeting. I pulled into Pleasant Valley's parking lot at precisely two o'clock, because I wanted to make sure that I arrived after lunch had finished but before dinner had begun, thus working around the undeviating regimen of mealtimes that regulates a resident's daily life. Indeed, the unremitting sameness of a resident's day-to-day routine, broken only by the occasional "activity" of a sing-a-long led by a piano-playing volunteer or of a bingo game run by some available staff member, necessitates virtually every SNF posting at or near its nurses' station a large sign informing residents of the current day, month, and year, together with the next upcoming holiday. Little wonder, then, that SNF residents can experience the passage of time the way prison inmates do—except that those incarcerated in penitentiaries have greater prospects of one day being released into the outside world.

As I walked up the sidewalk from Pleasant Valley's parking lot, I noticed in front of the main-entrance's double doors a bench not present the week before. Perhaps, I thought, a SNF administrator or family member had placed it there, feeling fresh air might do the residents some good. But no resident sat upon the bench—only a SNF worker on her break smoking a cigarette. I walked past her into the facility and once more began the drill: I pressed my way between the wheelchairs abutting the main desk, wrote my name down in the log, showed my ID badge to a different nurse (who nonetheless responded with yet-another "Hello, Doctor! What can I do for you?"), got hold of Lucille's chart, and lightly browsed the intervening week's progress notes left by the SNF's staff as well as by our hospice's. As I had done the first time I saw Lucille, when I finished with her chart, I tucked it on the ledge beneath the countertop so I could easily retrieve it on my way back out.

Veering around the various serving trays, med carts, and wheelchairs scattered throughout the corridors, I eventually came to Lucille's hallway and worked my way down to the last room on it. As always, I knocked prior to going in: "Lucille, it's Michael Goldberg. May I come in?"

"Hold on a minute! I wasn't expecting you today!"

Nor had she any reason to. SNF hospice patients with slow declines like hers—and with daily schedules and whereabouts that typically never vary—normally don't get the firmly-scheduled appointments generally given other hospice patients still living in their own homes, but who might have shorter-term, more crisis-ridden prognoses. In that regard, even hospice chaplaincy, like the rest of healthcare, triages its resources.

"You can come in now," I heard her say after a few moments.

"Glad to see you again, Lucille," I said as I stepped into her room. "And your smile looks better than ever!"

"Why, thank you. I can't tell you how much better these new choppers make me feel about myself."

Even though Lucille's chart indicated she could still get around with a walker, yet there she lay in bed before me, the same as the week before. For all I knew, she never left the bed. More bluntly put, I wondered whether the staff so much as ever offered her any help to leave it.

"You know," I ventured, "it's a beautiful day, and as I was entering the lobby, I noticed a new bench out front. I thought maybe we could go outdoors and sit for a while. Have you been up and around yet?"

"To tell the truth, no. I'd like to get out of this bed more than I do, but they simply don't have enough staff here to attend to each and every one of us, and it takes time to get me up and dressed."

"Then how about this, Lucille? When I come by next Wednesday *at this same time*, why don't we plan on going outside?"

"I would enjoy that very much. I haven't been asked out on a date in years!"

Once more, she smiled. New teeth alone couldn't account for a smile like that.

"Lucille," I said, "both times I've come by, I've noticed how cheerful you seem. How do you do it?"

"I've never really thought about it. Life is what it is. My father died when I was fourteen, and I had to help my mother raise my younger sister and brother. By the time I was nineteen, I was married with one child already and with another on the way. My husband, Jack, was a good, kind man, who worked forty years as a toolmaker to support our family. Not that I wasn't a good wife! He would come home from work every day at four o'clock and want sex, and no matter how tired I was, I made sure he got it—followed by dinner promptly at six. Keeping the boys out of the house in the late afternoon but still getting them back home in time to eat took some planning, believe you me!"

I found myself momentarily taken aback by Lucille's frankness; despite the clinical setting and my training, I felt as though I were listening to my grandmother's talking about her marital relations with my grandfather. But the very humor and nonchalance with which Lucille recounted her life story put me at ease, leaving me eager to hear more.

"After the boys grew up, Jack and I sold our house and moved into a condominium. After he died, I continued living there for several years by myself. I kept my old 'lady-friends,' even made some new ones, and we did what women our age did—went out to lunch, gossiped, went to movies, gossiped, went shopping, and gossiped. I didn't like being alone, but I really didn't have much choice. My sons didn't invite me to come live with them, and no man asked me to marry him. As the years passed, most of my friends began to move away or die. Then, about three or four years ago, I had a few accidents—you know, a couple of falls, some fainting spells. After that, Brian and Phil persuaded me to give up the condo and move in here. It wasn't and isn't easy, but what can you do? Life is life."

"Even so," I said, "life consists of lots and lots of days and each of those days contains lots and lots more hours. What do you do to pass the time here?"

"I try to make friends with the staff. Most of them can hardly speak English. But there is one little Filipino aide who works here who is very bright. She goes to a community college. I help her with her homework, and she plays Scrabble with me." Lucille opened her nightstand's single drawer and took out a miniature Scrabble set.

"I'd be glad to play a game with you," I volunteered, thinking I might have struck upon a sure-fire way to give her more of the camaraderie she so obviously desired.

"Are you any good?" she asked.

"Well, I haven't played for quite a while, but I still remember the rules, I think."

"No, thanks," she snorted, quickly shutting the game back into the nightstand. "I used to be a champion—I don't like playing with amateurs."

Feeling that my offer had been dismissed unfairly, I responded some-what defensively, "But what about the aide you play with?"

"That girl is the exception, and I say that not merely because she's bright and I like her. It's one of the few ways of getting some attention around here."

"Alright, I get it about Scrabble," I said, my bruised ego having been somewhat assuaged by Lucille's explanation. "But is there something else I can do for you today to keep you company?"

"Yes, you have a soothing voice. Would you mind reading to me for a while?" Lucille took a year-old copy of *Reader's Digest* from atop the nightstand and handed it to me. "Start reading anywhere. It really doesn't matter." Five minutes later, when I looked up, she was sound asleep.

My rounds ended sooner that afternoon than I had anticipated. Two patients called to cancel their appointments, and in recent weeks, the hospice's patient census and thus my own had both dropped dramatically. With no remaining patients left to see that day, I decided to head back to the office to catch up on my phone calls and complete some unfinished paperwork.

Ordinarily, the hospice office wouldn't have provided me space for doing either. Small to begin with, it had been subdivided into a dozen constricted cubicles, whose tabletops were separated from one another by flimsy plastic panels, akin to carpeted pizza slices. Moreover, only half the cubicles had phones, and normally, they would have been in use by nurses and aides from early morning through mid-afternoon. But by half past four, the office had all but emptied out. I found a cubicle with a phone and pushed "9" to get an outside line in another attempt to reach Lucille's son, Brian. Both the SNF's chart and our own had listed him as her "DPOAHC," that is, as the person holding her "Durable Power of Attorney for Health Care."

"Hello?" answered a beleaguered-sounding voice at the other end.

"Hello, this is Michael Goldberg, and I'm with Wellspring Hospice. I'd like to speak with Brian Larkin." Besides once again wishing to protect Lucille's privacy, I wanted to avoid, at least initially, identifying myself as "the chaplain." While some family members too readily associate *any* call from "hospice" with bad news, others too hastily equate one from "the chaplain" with news of death itself.

The voice at the other end grew more agitated: "Speaking!"

"As I was saying, Mr. Larkin, my name is Michael Goldberg, and I'm with Wellspring Hospice," I repeated, trying to remain pleasant despite Brian's asperity. "I serve on the staff as a chaplain, and I've been visiting your mother. I saw her earlier today, in fact, and all things considered, she appears to be holding her own both physically and emotionally."

I hoped that my having provided Brian with a fresh update about his mother might open him up to giving me some more information about her past. Brian's response, however, instantly scotched such hopes: "Anything else? I've got to go."

If Brian wanted to speak to me as though I were a telemarketer, then I would try to keep him on the line until I got what I wanted—or until he hung up on me outright. What did I have to lose?

"I'll try to keep it short then, Mr. Larkin," I continued. "Hospice alleviates physical suffering at the end of life through its expert administration of pain medications. Adequately relieving psychic suffering can be much harder, though. On that score, your mother gives me one specific area of concern. She's told me she wishes she had more company. To her credit, she's reached out to some of the facility's staff members, put in a request for a hospice volunteer to visit her, and asked me to continue to come by regularly, which, of course, I'm glad to do. During the time I'm with her, I'd naturally like to do things she might enjoy. Can you suggest any? Today, for instance, she mentioned that she was a former Scrabble champion. And yet, when I offered to play a game of it with her, she turned me down cold."

Brian's voice rose in anger. "Typical! She's so manipulative! Believe me, the more you get to know her, the more you'll understand why she's so alone! Nobody's *ever* good enough for her. Near-term, I can't foresee any flexibility in my schedule permitting me to fly out to see her. Let me know when she's near the end: I'll try to make some time to fly out then. Like I said, I've got to go." The line went dead. Brian had, indeed, hung up.

I had no idea what lay beneath the rage Brian harbored toward his mother, but I had a sense Phil might. Equally important, I thought that since Phil lived only one state away, he might consider paying Lucille a visit sometime sooner, at least, than Brian. I called him and recited the same self-introduction I had given Brian, along with the same update about their mother.

Phil, unlike Brian, responded in a gentle and empathetic voice, and of greatest significance for my work trying to help Lucille, in a manner that provided new pieces of her life story.

"Gosh, Chaplain, I'm sorry, but not surprised, by what you've said about Mother's current situation. Throughout her life, she was always surrounded by people. When she was in her early teens, her father died, and our grandmother increasingly relied on her to take care of her little sister and brother. I can remember Mother telling us how demanding Grandmother was with her! Anyway, by the time she had reached her late teens, Mother had gotten married and had had Brian and me in short succession. Even after our father's death and our moving out of the house, she still had her network of friends, women's clubs, and church groups. So you see, she's never really even had a chance to be alone until fairly late into her life."

Phil had given me some insight into Lucille's need for companion-ship. But he still hadn't told me why Brian's relationship with their mother seemed so strained. However, I didn't want to offend Phil by appearing critical of his brother in any way.

"Brian seemed a bit rushed when I called him," I said. "You know him far, far better than I do. Are there better times to reach him?"

"Chaplain, I'm afraid that when it comes to talking about Mother, there are no good times for Brian. He has such mixed feelings toward her. She certainly gave Brian the push to succeed. But sometimes, she might have pushed too hard. Me, she didn't push at all. Maybe that's why Brian is a top-level executive at a Fortune 500 company in New York, and why I'm a used-car salesman here in Phoenix. I guess Mother raised Brian and me the way Grandmother raised her and her younger siblings: demand a lot from the oldest child, and as far as any other child, whatever happens, happens."

As Phil fleshed out the Larkin family history, he spoke without a shred of regret or resentment, and as a result, I felt on safe ground raising the issue of greatest import to Lucille's spiritual well-being: "Phil, do you have any plans to come visit your mother sometime soon?"

"No, Chaplain, I don't. But please keep me updated about her condition—especially if she doesn't have much time left." Except for Phil's saying, "Please," I might as well have been talking with Brian.

I thanked Phil, hung up, wrote separate summaries of my conversations with him and Brian, and along with my written request for a volunteer, placed everything in the folder our office had set aside for any new documentation on Lucille. In addition, I jotted down a reminder to myself to bring a more recent *Reader's Digest* on my next visit, together with a word game Lucille might play with me instead of Scrabble.

Thus, when I returned to Pleasant Valley, I came fully equipped with a new magazine and game. After yet again running the gauntlet of the SNF's *pro formas* from log-in to ID-display to staff-greeting to chart-check (interspersed, of course, with the apparently inexorable "Hello, Doctor!"), I bounded down the halls to the last room on Lucille's corridor. But the second I went inside and saw her, I knew something was horribly wrong: she lay in her bed ashen-faced and trembling. I put down the magazine and game and pulled out my cell phone, prepared to make an emergency call to a hospice nurse.

"Lucille, what is it?" I asked, trying to keep my voice and manner calm so as not to upset her further.

"I've been trying to get somebody to come for over an hour," she whimpered.

"Are you in pain?"

"No, I just don't like being alone. The longer it lasts, the more anxious I get, until finally, it becomes unbearable."

I took her hand. "It's OK now. I'm here with you, and I'll stay here as long as you need me to. Look: I even brought a new magazine for me to read to you and a new word game, Boggle, for you and me to play."

"Thank you," she said as she started to relax. "I guess I'm even dressed for the occasion. I've already got my dentures in."

"I'm glad. Why don't we go outside for a little air, then? Let me look for an aide with a wheelchair. I'll only be gone for a minute or two."

Lucille smiled, and I left her room to find an aide with a wheelchair. Seeing nobody in the hall and not wanting to leave Lucille alone for long, I started walking briskly, almost running, up to where her corridor met the next. Down at that hallway's other end, I spied a lone aide whom I hoped might mistake me for a physician yet one more time. "Excuse me," I called," I need someone to help Ms. Larkin get out of her bed and into a wheelchair."

The aide didn't even look up at me. Whether physician, chaplain, or even the Almighty, she couldn't have cared less who was addressing her. "She's not one of my patients," the aide said indifferently. "I couldn't even tell you which room or bed she's in."

"OK, then," I retorted with more than a tinge of irritation, "I'll be glad to show you."

With that, the aided looked up, scowled, went inside a resident's room, and came out with a wheelchair that she started pushing up the hallway toward me. For my part, I began walking back rapidly to Lucille's room, glancing over my shoulder repeatedly to make sure the aide was staying close behind. By the time we managed to return to Lucille, however, the color from her face had drained completely, and her trembling had recommenced full-force. Only a fleeting smile that washed across her face upon seeing me reflected any sign of relief at all.

Sullenly, the aide sat Lucille on the edge of her bed, pushed the wheelchair next to her, and, after having hoisted her up, slid her down inside it. I thanked the aide for her assistance. She glared at me, turned, and left.

I rolled Lucille out to Pleasant Valley's front lawn. She couldn't remember, she told me, when she had last been outside. We chatted a while, and then I read a few articles from the *Reader's Digest* I had brought, having plucked both it and the word game off her nightstand as we had left her room. News of a certain celebrity couple's break-up struck her as a bombshell: she didn't even know they had gotten married two years before. An hour or so later, she said she was getting chilled and asked me to take her back indoors. I assumed she wanted to go back to bed, but instead, she wished only to go back inside Pleasant Valley's lobby, saying that she'd like to play my new word game, Boggle. Unlike Scrabble, Boggle hinges on a player's ability not merely to form individual letters into words, but to do so quickly before the sands in a tiny hour-glass run out. I figured that my being several decades Lucille's junior would give me a distinct advantage. I was wrong. Although I won the first game—Lucille had, after all, never previously played Boggle—she bested me every game thereafter. "It's OK," she kidded, "if you practice for about ten years' more, you'll have another chance to beat me. Of course, from what the doctors tell me, you've really only got about six months to ratchet up your game a notch."

We spent about another half an hour talking until, finally tiring, she said, "Our big day on the town has taken the starch out of me. Could you please take me back to my room?" Obligingly, I put my weight behind her chair to start rolling it down the series of passageways awaiting us when suddenly, Lucille grabbed its wheels to stop me.

"Michael, I'd like you to leave me here at the nurses' station. At least I'll have some people around me. I don't tend to get the jitters as much as when I'm all alone."

"I understand," I said as I wheeled her chair close against the main desk. Then, I leaned over, hugged her, and whispered, "Lucille, from now on, I'll be here to see you the same day, the same time, each and every week. I give you my word." She smiled up at me—and she kept smiling at me as I completed my procedures for logging out, pushed open Pleasant Valley's double doors, and stepped into its parking lot.

One more piece of work, however, awaited me at Pleasant Valley before I drove away. I needed to inform the SNF's chief administrator of Lucille's condition when I had first arrived. I hadn't wanted to go searching for him, though, within eyesight of Lucille, fearing I might somehow disturb her new-found equilibrium. Thus, once inside my car, I got him on my cell phone. I reported to him, as politely but as firmly as I could, that as a result of his staff's failure to respond to Lucille's repeated calls for help, she had suffered a panic attack lasting well over an hour. But the administrator's responsiveness proved as wanting as any of his subordinates': "Old people just get confused when it comes to things like time." "Oh, *really*?" I thought to myself. "Have *you* ever sat down with Ms. Larkin to play a game of Boggle?"

I said goodbye as courteously as I could manage under the circumstances and immediately called the hospice. I got patched through to Rose, one of the nurses fielding calls. When I reported Lucille's panic attack and its cause, she asked me to wait while she pulled up Lucille's computer file.

"Michael," Rose said, "Ms. Larkin's medications already include Ativan p.r.n." Ativan, a highly-effective anti-anxiety drug,[7] is routinely given hospice patients at their request, or "p.r.n."—short for the Latin, *pro re nata*, which means, in fact, precisely that: "*when needed*." But how could Lucille get the SNF's personnel to respond to her need for Ativan when, given my experience with them thus far, they seemed so unresponsive to *any* of her needs?

The next week, I drove back to Pleasant Valley for my appointment with Lucille. I went through the obligatory check-in drill at the front desk and walked swiftly through the various passageways that led to the corridor at whose foot stood Room 42. I entered Lucille's room, only to discover bed B empty. I quickly stuck my head around the curtain to ask "the moaner" if she knew where Lucille might be. But her bed, too, lay vacant. A single thought raced across my mind—both residents were dead. I glanced down at my watch. Since lunchtime had passed a couple hours ago, no residents would continue to occupy the dining room. Only one more place remained to look for her: the activities room.

"It's the man from hostage!" Lucille cried out to no one in particular as she saw me come through the activities room door. A misnomer if ever there were one, the "activities room" stood devoid of any goings-on, either organized or unstructured. Its "furnishings" featured a scarred piano pushed up against one wall, a dozen battered folding chairs leaning on another, and some pictures that might qualify as kindergarten "art projects" taped indiscriminately to the other two. Besides Lucille, several residents (including "the moaner") sat idly in their wheelchairs, aimlessly strewn about, while a solitary aide hunched over a supermarket tabloid, turning its pages absently. I felt enormous relief when I saw that both Lucille and her sense of humor still remained alive. But when I pulled up a chair and started to sit down next to her, I saw something that filled me with distress once more. As Lucille smiled, her grin resembled an upturned hot-dog bun with its edges—her lips!—curled inwards, her mouth now altogether toothless, looking as though it belonged on a mask fit solely for a Halloween witch's fright face.

"Michael," she exclaimed before I could even fully take my seat, "somebody stole my teeth!"

"What do you mean 'stole'?"

---

7. Known generically as "Lorazepam."

"You heard me: '*stole*'!"

To my knowledge, no black market existed, inside the nursing home or out, for custom-fitted dentures. But I could easily believe things got routinely lost at Pleasant Valley.

"Lucille, maybe somebody accidentally misplaced them."

All traces of any kind of smile instantly vanished from her face. "Michael, do *you* think I'm senile?"

"No, that's not what I meant!" I didn't want Lucille to think for a moment I shared the SNF administrator's point of view concerning the elderly and their bouts of "confusion."

"Well, the people here are treating me like one more little old lady who has lost her marbles. I don't know what happened to my dentures. Maybe they weren't stolen. But I didn't simply 'lose' them. Can you help me?"

"I don't know Lucille, but I'll do what I can."

Lucille and I spent only a brief bit time more together before she asked me to wheel her back to her room. Her frustration with the staff's lack of responsiveness in helping her locate her dentures, combined with her self-consciousness over her appearance, outweighed her desire for company. Knowing how prone she could be to anxiety, I didn't want to take a chance on roiling her further by facilely attempting to change the subject.

Later that day, I called Kirsten, the hospice social worker assigned to Lucille's case, to tell her about the missing dentures.

"Yes, Michael, I already know all about it," Kirsten replied. "Lucille brought it up first thing when I met with her last Friday."

"So what do you think happened to her teeth?" I asked.

Kirsten paused a moment before answering. "In the course of a SNF's daily routine of taking care of both its residents and the physical facility itself, things do go missing—though not generally due to any malice or criminal activity. You know how it is, Michael. The people who work there are understaffed and overtasked, and some of the residents are genuinely forgetful."

"But what about Lucille specifically, Kirsten?" I pressed. "Would you call *her* 'forgetful'?"

"Not in the slightest!"

"So, then," I continued, "how do we go about finding her old set of dentures, or, failing that, getting her a new replacement set?"

"Getting her a new pair is going to be tough," Kirsten replied. "Under Medicare rules, she's only allowed one new pair every five years."

"What?!" I erupted. "She'd be ninety-three! I know she's on hospice, but given her diagnosis, she could live lots longer than six months. What's she supposed to eat for the rest of her life? Green gruel through a straw?!"

The social worker in Kirsten took over. "Calm down, Michael. Why don't we try to resolve Lucille's problem together? First, I'll talk with the SNF's administrator to see if I can't get him to have the staff do a more thorough search for Lucille's missing teeth. After that, I'll speak with her sons—although I don't expect much help from either one of them; there are too many family issues. While I'm working on the problem from those angles, why don't you put in a call to Twyla to find out if we've got any connections with dentists willing to volunteer their services to make Lucille some new dentures, just in case?"

Both Kirsten and I knew that we were pursuing long shots. As a result, neither of us was surprised when the administrator adamantly insisted that his staff would never simply lose, much less steal, a pair of dentures; if Lucille's teeth had disappeared, the source, he reiterated, lay in the "confusion" typical of those of her advanced age. But Kirsten persisted until the administrator grudgingly ordered one more search for Lucille's teeth. Afterwards, Kirsten called me and left a message: "One of the SNF aides took all of five minutes looking for the dentures in Lucille's nightstand and under her bed. Guess what? She didn't find anything. No surprise there. I hope you have better luck with Twyla."

I didn't. Twyla told me that although she empathized with Lucille's situation, the hospice didn't have any connections with free or low-cost dental services. "I wish we did," she said. "We're running into increasing numbers of older patients with significant dental problems. I don't think evolution intended our teeth to last us as long as we're generally living nowadays."

Kirsten, Twyla, and I had tried our best. But although I couldn't get Lucille new dentures, I could still give her ongoing companionship. Over the next five months, I kept visiting her regularly, always arriving at our pre-agreed upon day and time. In the beginning, some things never changed during those visits: weather permitting, I'd wheel her outdoors; I'd hear her past week's "news"; I'd read to her; we'd play Boggle—she'd *always* win. As time wore on, however, two things changed noticeably for the worse: her weight and mood. Without her teeth, Lucille's diet consisted of two unappealing choices, either Ensure—which she detested as "Wheaties for Old Folks"—or whatever puree the SNF's kitchen could concoct. Not surprisingly, Lucille found the unvarying daily menu bland and unappetizing, and consequently, whatever its purported nutritional value, she took in less and less of the liquid fare set before her. As her weight dropped and her strength declined, her anxiety intensified. Her once-easy smile utterly disappeared, and she increasingly passed our time together without a word, not wanting to leave her bed or let go my hand.

Then one day, as I walked into her room, she looked up at me and flashed a wide smile chock-full of teeth.

"Lucille!" I blurted out in astonishment. "Where on earth did you get those teeth?"

"I finally called Brian and told him, 'Dammit! I need you and Phil to buy me a new set of false teeth.' I hated to have to do it, but I couldn't down one more gulp of the kitchen's swill."

Why, I wondered, hadn't Lucille turned to her sons earlier? An unwillingness to "impose"? A fear of possible rejection? Something to do, perhaps, with the "family issues" to which Kirsten had earlier alluded? But why, then, had Brian (and Phil?) come through now? Maybe here, near the end of Lucille's life, earlier hard feelings had finally softened and given way to reconciliation.

Lucille and I chatted comfortably for well over an hour. Then I read to her for another thirty minutes. Finally, we played a game of Boggle, which (of course) she won. I said my farewells, logged out, and went to my car to call Brian, filled with curiosity about what had so unexpectedly motivated him and Phil to come to their mother's aid.

"Hello, Mr. Larkin, this is Michael Goldberg, the chaplain from Wellspring Hospice. I've just left your mother, and she looks so much better, physically and emotionally. Those teeth you and Phil got her have made a world of difference!"

"Phil didn't contribute anything toward buying them," bristled Brian. "Anyway, if those dentures will keep her quiet for a while, then they're worth every cent. It's one less distraction in my life." Then, after pausing a few seconds, he asked, "How much longer do you think she's got?"

Ironically, my answer might not have been the one most welcome from Brian's perspective. "Now that she can eat solid food again and has regained her spirits, she's showing some marked improvement." Then I quickly added, wary of Brian's inclination summarily to cut me off, "Since your mother's feeling a little better at the moment, you might want to take the opportunity to fly out here and see her."

I heard nothing but silence on the line. Finally, Brian said, "I'm pretty busy now. I'll try and make it later—when she's at the end." Then, as before, he just hung up.

I put a call into Phil. I might as well have been hitting the "replay" button of my talk with Brian: "Too many balls in the air to come see Mother now. But let me know when we're near the end."

Three months passed. Finally, despite her winning smile, despite her humor, despite *herself,* Lucille's decline in body as well as spirit became more and more apparent. True to her diagnosis, she was indeed "failing to thrive." Kirsten and I each made repeated calls to Brian and Phil, urging them to come to their mother's bedside while she still possessed the ability to interact with them, that it looked as if the end were in fact nearing. The response we received from each brother remained unchanged: "Call me when she's *really* dying; *then* I'll come." Kirsten and I concluded Lucille might well never see either of her sons again.

The two of us, however, kept on visiting Lucille and providing her with what companionship we could. But each visit became briefer as Lucille tired more easily and fell asleep more quickly. The day came when she lost to me at Boggle a second time. "Don't gloat," she jibed. "You only beat an old dying lady." Eventually, conversations with her became limited to single words, bracketed by long periods of quiet. Death was drawing closer every day.

Then one afternoon I had only to walk through Pleasant Valley's double doors to find Lucille and see that something was dreadfully wrong with her. She sat in her wheelchair parked up against the main nurses' station as her body shook violently, wracked, I suspected, by the same unbearable anxiety I had witnessed months before when her unheeded calls for Ativan—and company—had ultimately overwhelmed her. Yet unlike then, now she had a nurse close by, barely a foot away behind the desk. Stranger still, no other resident, wheelchair-bound or otherwise, occupied the lobby. As I moved forward to put my hand on Lucille's and lean down to speak with her, the nurse behind the desk abruptly swung around it and thrust herself in front of me.

"Oh, Doctor! [*Still,* after all my visits!] What perfect timing! State inspectors showed up ten minutes ago for a surprise visit, and they view our having residents sitting around the lobby as some sort of fire-safety issue. So we've returned all the residents to their rooms—all except Lucille, that is. As you can see for yourself, she's having another of her fits. But leaving her alone in her room hollering for help won't make us look good, either. Would you mind having a word with her to quiet her down so we can get her back in bed?"

For once, I was willing to let the SNF staff call me "Doctor" without correction. "Has anybody given Ms. Larkin her Ativan? Look at her chart. It's p.r.n."

"No, we've been so busy getting the residents back to their rooms," replied the nurse, "we haven't had the time."

"Fine. I'll wheel Ms. Larkin back to 42B," I said, making a point of Lucille's location. "Meanwhile, you send somebody down there with her meds—*stat*. Agreed?"

"Yes, Doctor."

The nurse turned away, and I approached Lucille, bent down, and said softly in her ear, "It's OK now, Lucille. I'm here, I'm taking you back to your room, and I'll stay with you until they bring you your Ativan." Lucille stared straight ahead, her body shuddering without cessation.

I rolled her wheelchair through the now nearly-deserted hallways, coming finally to the foot of hers, where I carefully eased her chair through the door leading into her room. Then, I took the lone chair inside the room and drew it next to her. As I began to sit down, Lucille grasped my hands. I tried to speak to her soothingly—about what I don't recall. I only remember half an hour's elapsing without any nurse's yet having brought Lucille her Ativan.

"Lucille," I lied, "sitting in this chair has given me a little spasm in my back. I feel like I need to stretch it out a tad against one of the walls in the corridor. Do you mind if I step out for a moment?"

I could barely hear her as she answered, "No."

I got up, peered out of the room and up the hall, and glimpsed a nurse with a med cart rounding the corner. Today of all days, what with the inspectors present, she would follow every drug-dispensing protocol to the letter. She would start with the first room at the top of the corridor and methodically work her way down the hallway to the room at its very end: Lucille's.

I strode hurriedly up the hall, ready to rely again on my alter ego and his cachet. "Nurse!" I called insistently.

"Yes, Doctor?"

"Ms. Larkin has been waiting for her Ativan for half an hour. She's very agitated, and as I told another nurse at the front desk when I first got here, you'll see in her chart that the Ativan is p.r.n." Then I caught myself lest, sounding imperious, I turn a merely tardy nurse into a resentful one whose appearance at 42B would come not sooner but, if possible, even later. "Would you please," I began again, "go down to her room and give her medication to her now?"

"Why, of course, Doctor."

"Greatly appreciated," I replied as I turned and retraced my steps back down to Lucille's room as fast as I could go. Even though I had been absent for two or three minutes at most, when I re-entered her room, I saw waves of shuddering again coursing through her body, now joined by a stream of panicked outcries spewing from her mouth: "I can't go on with trying to figure out this world! I'm lost! Brian is lost, and Phil is lost! There is no peace here! My God, there is no meaning here—everything you touch is meaningless!"

"Lucille, I'm back," I said trying to calm her. "Don't worry. The nurse will be here any second with your Ativan."

"Any second" might as well have meant "any century." After waiting another fifteen minutes while attempting, without success, to ease Lucille's anxiety, I once again excused myself, slipped out into the hallway, and took a few steps up the corridor hunting for the nurse. Neither she—nor her med cart—was anywhere in sight. I didn't want to leave Lucille to go searching for them. And even if I found the nurse, what could I do then? Haul her by her arm back to Lucille's room and force her to give Lucille the medication? I went back inside Lucille's room, sat down beside her, and stroked her hair for the next half hour. It seemed to work: her breathing slowed, her trembling stopped, and she appeared at ease once more.

Suddenly, my pager chirped. Automatically, I reached inside my pants to throttle it, worried that its noise might startle Lucille and set her off anew. But once I had pulled the pager out and read it, I knew nothing could alarm Lucille more than the message it displayed: "Return to office immediately."

Once more, I had to excuse myself and step out into the hallway. I walked a few yards up the corridor so that Lucille couldn't hear me, and bracing my body against a wall, I called the office on my cell phone.

"Wellspring Hospice, how may I help you?" asked Lana, the receptionist.

"Lana, this is Michael. I got a page a few seconds ago to return to the office immediately."

"Michael, *everybody* has been paged to come in."

"Why? What's wrong?"

"It's Janine," Lana answered, referring to our hospice's general manager. "The budget numbers came in today, and I guess they don't look good. Janine wants to talk with the whole staff ASAP about improving them. She sounds really frantic."

Janine, like many hospice administrators, had begun her career as an RN, later taken some management courses, and over the years risen through the ranks of our non-profit hospice's "business side." And make no mistake. Nonprofit hospices, just like for-profit ones, have a business side: for both kinds, if their expenses exceed their incomes, their demise is as inevitable as any of their patients.

I asked Lana to patch me through to Janine. "Hello, Michael. What is it?" Janine said, her words even more clipped than usual.

"Janine, even as we speak, one of our long-time SNF patients, Ms. Lucille Larkin, is undergoing a severe panic attack. Our patient's chart says that she is to have Ativan p.r.n., but I can't get any SNF personnel to bring it to her. Our patient has no family living locally, and she may be nearing death. I've been waiting with Ms. Larkin in her room, because being left alone only increases our patient's suffering." In repeatedly referring to Lucille as "*our* patient," I wanted to emphasize to Janine our hospice's responsibility to provide care for Lucille, especially during such a crisis.

But to Janine, whether Lucille was our patient or somebody else's ultimately made no difference. "Well, Michael," she replied, "that's unfortunate, but you still have to come in. I need to meet with you and the other staff for a talk on 'Hospice Economics 101.' Unless you all begin to pay better attention to our financials, not only won't we be able to help *this* patient, we won't be able to help *any* patients. See you in an hour. Goodbye."

When I looked down at my cell phone to flip it shut, I saw that my own hand was now shaking as violently as Lucille's whole body had been less than half an hour ago. But whereas Lucille's trembling had been sparked by anxiety, mine had been ignited by rage: at the med-cart nurse, at Janine, at my own powerlessness. I stuck my hand inside my pocket so that Lucille wouldn't see it when I went back into her room.

"Lucille," I said meekly, "I returned the page from my office, and they told me I have to drive back there right away."

"Please don't leave me," she begged.

"Lucille, I'm so sorry, but I have to go. On my way out, I'll look for the med-cart nurse to bring you the Ativan. Is the young aide you befriended working here today? Maybe I could send her down," I said, fishing for some way to make my departure easier on both of us.

"No," Lucille answered as she gazed down at her slippers on the wheelchair's footrests. "She's on vacation—gone back to the Philippines for a month to visit with her family."

"I'm truly sorry, Lucille," I mumbled yet again. Then I leaned over and hugged her and turned away. As I left her room, I heard her crying. The farther up the corridor I walked, the louder it seemed to get.

As I made my may through the SNF's hallways, not a single nurse or aide came into view; they were all attending to the residents inside their rooms, perhaps trying to keep out of sight of the probing eyes of the state inspectors as well as out of earshot of any prying questions they might pose. Only at the nurses' station by the front entrance did I come across a staff member, the same nurse who had asked me to wheel Lucille back to her room close to two hours earlier. Desperate to get Lucille her Ativan— and maybe in the process even a few minutes' company—I held up my hospice badge to within inches of the nurse's face, thus relinquishing any chance of her ever again mistaking me for a doctor. "Please," I pleaded with the nurse, "Ms. Larkin in 42B hasn't calmed down since you last saw her almost two hours ago. It's been forty-five minutes since a med-cart nurse promised me she would bring Ms. Larkin her Ativan, but she still hasn't come. I've been waiting with Ms. Larkin the entire time. Now, I've been paged elsewhere." Then, as if to underscore both my entreaty and its urgency, I implored the nurse again, "*Please* send someone down to give Lucille her meds."

"I don't know," the nurse said blankly. "I've got a lot on my hands."

I walked through Pleasant Valley's double doors, got into my car, and headed back to the hospice office to hear Janine lecture us on being more cost-effective.

The next morning, I checked my voicemail to pick up messages about my patients. The first came from the on-call nurse: "Lucille Larkin died last night at 10:30 PM." Missing from the message was the phrase that typically accompanies notification of virtually every hospice patient's passing: "Her death was a peaceful one."

"From your experience," people sometimes ask me, "what's the worst possible way to die?" I don't have to think twice about my answer: alone.

7

Cheryl's Torso

HAVING MOVED ON TO work with a different hospice in Southern California, I exited yet another gray slab of Los Angeles freeway and then drove past block after block of strip malls with facades the color of terracotta pancake makeup before I finally arrived at a cluster of faux-Tudor condominiums within whose warren of buildings and breezeways my new patient, according to the intake notes, somewhere resided. But the complex's gated garage barred my entry, forcing me to drive to the first available onstreet parking space, nearly half a mile away. I swung my briefcase with its bundle of documentation forms over the car's backseat, got out, and started trudging back. The calendar may have shown the date as sometime in early March, but the air in the San Fernando Valley had the feel and look of a day in late July, warm and humid beneath an ochre cupola of smog.

After about fifteen minutes, I reached the complex—only to discover another lengthy hike awaiting me, thanks, in no small measure, to the "assistance" proffered by some of the property's other tenants: "You're close! Building G is about four or five buildings over!"; "Oh no! G is *that* way!"; "Turn around, go back the way you've come, and you'll run right into G!" After traipsing back and forth for almost twenty minutes more, I stood at last in front of a door, with "2G" painted in Old English script beside it. I had not yet knocked, when from inside, a woman's voice rang out, "Who's there?"

"Michael Goldberg from Caritas Hospice."

The door slowly opened to reveal not so much the thirty-year-old woman of the intake notes as a spindle, atop which sat a long, thin face, encased by straight, black hair. "I heard you coming to the door. Come on in. I'm Cheryl Wolfe, the one who, in case you couldn't tell, is dying."

I entered a home within whose likes I had set foot too many times before, when visiting other hospice patients: its shades were drawn as though sunlight served as an excessively harsh reminder of life's continuation in the world beyond. Cheryl led me the few steps to the living room where, as my eyes adjusted to the darkness, I could discern the outlines of two figures seated on a sofa. One looked to be a man roughly about Cheryl's age, the other an older woman who, as soon as I came within her range, bleated out at me, "What's wrong with you hospice people? Don't you know how sick Cheryl is? We've been expecting the nurse for hours!"

"I'm sorry, Ma'am," I began, "I'll be glad to call the office—"

"Dammit, Ma!" Cheryl cut in, "It's only 2:00! Remember? Their nurse, Billie, isn't supposed to get here until 3:30. And besides, I'm OK right now—no pain, no nausea, no nothing."

The young man, perhaps embarrassed by the outbursts of mother and daughter alike and hence eager to distract me, got up quickly off the couch, strode over, and thrust out his hand. "Hi, I'm Marc Lanier. Cheryl, Helen, and I were just having some tea. Can I offer you any? Or is there something else you'd prefer instead?" As Marc emerged from the shadows, a short, soft-featured man came into view, wisps of light brown hair ringing his balding head. Attired in "business casual," he sported tasseled loafers, pleated khaki slacks, and a blue, button-down shirt, open at the neck.

"No thanks, Marc," I replied. "It's nice to meet all of you. I'm glad to be of service in whatever way—"

Once again, Cheryl cut me off. "OK, I need to know two things. First, are you a rabbi? Second, do you perform weddings?"

"'Yes' on both counts," I responded.

"What about for hospice patients?"

"To be honest, I've never conducted a marriage in the course of my hospice work. None of my patients has ever requested it."

"Well, I might be the first one then," she crowed. "How would you feel about marrying Marc and me?"

Unprepared for Cheryl's directness, I stalled for time. "As with any prospective couple, I'd want to know more about you before agreeing." But my response made Cheryl only push harder. "OK, once you got to know us better, then what? Would you marry us after that?" I could see that she would not be easily dissuaded, and besides, performing weddings for my patients certainly fell within my job description of providing them spiritual support. "Sure, Cheryl," I answered, "all things being equal, I'd be glad to marry Marc and you."

"Good!" Cheryl said exultantly as though she had just closed some business deal. "Marc already has his own rabbi lined up to marry us, but I want to make certain we have a back-up if we need one."

Although slightly deflating, my relegation to second-stringer status nevertheless opened the door to my asking some questions of first-order importance for better acquainting myself with the couple and their history, both singly and together. "So, Marc," I inquired, "who exactly is your rabbi? Maybe I know him. I've lived in LA, on and off, for more than thirty years."

Marc's face lit up. "He's Rabbi Hershel Slatkin of Congregation Ner Tamid, and he's held the pulpit there for decades. Would you believe it? He '*bar mitzvahed*' me! Truth to tell, though, like many Jews, I stopped going to *shul*[1] shortly after that. But then, one Friday night after Cheryl got sick, I felt a need to go to services. Rabbi Slatkin somehow managed to pick me out in the crowd and amazingly, he remembered who I was. He came up to me at the *oneg*,[2] and since then, he's provided tremendous support not only to me, but to Cheryl and Helen as well. He's a wonderful man." From what I knew of Marc's rabbi, I liked him, too; by day's end, I would phone him, both as a courtesy and, in line with hospice protocol, as a way of coordinating whatever care we might plan on rendering.

"Your Rabbi Slatkin sounds like a real *mensch*,"[3] I said, echoing Marc's sentiments. Then in an attempt to elicit more of Marc's story from him, I added, "From what you've told me so far, I get the impression that you've spent most, if not all, of your life as an Angelino."

"That's right, Rabbi. I grew up out here in the Valley, and after high school, I went to UCLA. I stayed there to get my CPA degree. I guess my whole life has been relatively uneventful"—Marc paused and drew a deep breath—"until now, that is, with Cheryl's illness."

Cheryl reached over and clasped his hand. "Yeah, who would have ever thought that a 'nice Jewish boy' like Marc would have ended up with

1. Yiddish for "synagogue."

2. Hebrew for "enjoyment [of Shabbat]"—hence, colloquially, the social hour following Friday evening services.

3. Yiddish for "exemplary human being."

a girl like me—somebody who has lived her life anywhere *but* on 'the straight and narrow'?"

Turning to Helen, she asked, "Ma, could you go to the kitchen and make a fresh kettle of tea? This pot is way too weak for me."

After her mother had left the room, Cheryl turned back toward me. "After you hear what I have to say, you'll understand why I asked Ma to step out for a few minutes.

"I grew up in New York. One day, when I was in second grade, my dad simply didn't come home from work. Who knows why Dad left? As you saw for yourself, Ma can get to be a bit much.

"Anyhow, from a pretty early age, I ended up having to take care of both of us. By the time I was a teenager, I had learned enough about the stock market to finagle a broker's license. I eventually did well enough with my investments to move out here to take advantage of some bigger opportunities in real estate. I brought Ma with me. She could never have survived in New York without me.

"Long story short, I passed the real estate exam, and after a while, my business took off. I had been living here for about six years when a friend of Marc's, who also happened to be a former client of mine, introduced the two of us at a Dodgers' game. Marc and I started going out, and after about three or four months, we got engaged last October. We planned to get married this April. But in December," she said, maintaining the same matter-of-fact tone she had used throughout, "they diagnosed me with pancreatic cancer."

I knew two things about pancreatic cancer. First, it typically killed patients within three to six months of diagnosis. Second, in its final stages, pancreatic cancer could, absent proper pain management, leave those patients in agony.

Marc began to speak rapidly, albeit barely above a whisper. "I need to say something, too, before Helen comes back with the tea. Cheryl's physical condition isn't the only thing currently affecting the timing of an April ceremony. Helen's financial condition also concerns me. I don't know how much time I'll need to get her affairs in good order for the future. You saw for yourself how fragile she is even with Cheryl still here. Can you imagine just how much she might need once Cheryl is gone?"

"I understand, Marc," I said, trying to reassure him.

"Well, believe me, Rabbi, lots of our closest friends and family members have told us they can't begin to understand why, given Cheryl's cancer, the two of us plan on getting married at all."

At that point, Cheryl virtually leapt back into the conversation. "Look, from what the oncologists have told me and from what I've read, I don't believe for a minute that I'm going to 'lick this cancer.' In my work, I couldn't afford to be a romantic, and I don't intend to become one now. Whatever success I've attained has come from my ability to deal with cold, hard facts. The same goes for Marc. And from our perspective, here are the facts that matter in terms of our getting married: Marc and I love each other; I'm going to die; and, as a result, Marc will go through lots of grief. So looking at those facts, Michael, why the hell shouldn't we at least experience the joy of a wedding—along with however much time we have left afterwards as a married couple?"

Just then, Helen came back with the tea. "Rabbi, have they laid out to you this crazy plan of theirs to get married? I don't understand any of it—and I definitely don't know how I'm going to get along without my Cheryl!"

"I've told you before, Helen," Marc said patiently, "I'm making all the arrangements to ensure that you'll be OK."

Cheryl, having apparently heard such exchanges between Helen and Marc before, broke in and asked me, "Is there anything else you need to know about us now? I'm getting tired, and I'm still expecting your nurse, Billie, later this afternoon."

"Nothing else at the moment, Cheryl. But would you mind my coming back to see you once a week? As I said earlier, I'd like to get to know you and Marc better, in case you do end up having me perform your wedding."

Cheryl pondered my proposal for a few moments. "The differences between Marc's background and mine also extend to our religious upbringing. Ma and I have never even considered belonging to a temple. But who knows? Keeping you in the loop might come in handy."

"OK, then," said Marc, "we'll see you again next week. If anything comes up before then, we'll get in touch." I said my goodbyes, Cheryl showed me out, and I started making my way back to the car.

Torrential downpours accompanied my return to Cheryl's the following week. Despite them, I wanted to arrive punctually lest Helen's penchant for panic trigger the cannonade of emotional explosions I had witnessed during my initial visit. Fortunately, this time I had my choice of several close-by parking spaces. I had barely reached the door when, as before, Cheryl opened it. When she led me into the living room everything, in fact, appeared exactly as it had before: shades still drawn, Marc and Helen still seated in the darkness, Helen still perseverating about Billie's purported lateness. Then, as if to re-enact our first meeting in its entirety, Cheryl cut straight to her agenda item for the day: "You do funerals, yeah?"

"Yes," I answered, "I have, as a hospice chaplain, done funerals in the past. But you should know in advance that I don't do them often. Preparing eulogies, leading services, and consoling mourners all take time. I don't want to sound cold, Cheryl, but since you haven't pulled any punches with me, I'll level with you, too. The more time I spend on burying the dead, the less time I have to care for those patients of mine still living."

"Look, Rabbi," Marc chimed in, "I'd really appreciate your helping us out here. Yesterday, I drove out to one of the Jewish cemeteries in town, Home of Eternity, and purchased plots for all of us. As I mentioned when we met you, I've grown close to Rabbi Slatkin over the past few months, but in all honesty, his age might make it hard for him, physically as well as emotionally, to do both the wedding *and* the funeral."

Perhaps unconsciously, Marc the CPA had tallied up Rabbi Slatkin's assets against his liabilities, only to perceive some deficit once Cheryl's life had been stricken from the ledger. But Marc's comparison of Rabbi Slatkin's resources with my own in terms of assisting him with Cheryl's funeral rested on false reckoning. For Marc had utterly failed to factor the amount to which I myself might be taxed, physically, emotionally, and spiritually, prior to Cheryl's passing in caring not only for her needs, but for his and Helen's also. As a result, he had no way of accurately estimating how depleted my own reserves might be even to attend Cheryl's funeral, much less to conduct it, wedding intervening or no. And yet, as I sat opposite him and Cheryl in their darkened living room, their demonstrated need for peace of mind at present trumped any hypotheticals I had about my own future state of mind. Reluctantly, I agreed to officiate at Cheryl's funeral.

"Terrific!" Marc announced with an air of achievement. "Another 'to-do' crossed off the list."

"OK, then, Cheryl," I said as I changed the subject, "now that we've got that matter settled, let me ask you a question I know everybody from hospice puts to you at the outset of every visit. On a scale ranking your pain from '1' to '10', with '1' standing for 'nonexistent' and '10' meaning 'unbearable', how would you rate your pain level right now?"

"Only about a '2.'"

"Fine, I'm glad to hear it. Update me, then, about what's happened since my last visit."

"What else? Wedding planning!" Cheryl exclaimed. As she ticked off the details, she smiled for the first time since I had met her. "Marc and I thought about getting a caterer, but because my circumstances won't allow us to set a firm date and time, we decided instead to ask Marc's family and some friends to stand ready at an instant's notice to pick up deli, drinks, and even a wedding cake, if possible. Beyond that, finding a wedding gown has topped my list: I'll be damned if I'm getting married in my bathrobe! I've looked for a dress several sizes smaller than my current one—I know that as I get sicker, I'll get thinner, too. Those saleswomen probably mistake me for some bride-to-be on a crash diet that will squeeze her into her wedding gown. Maybe I'll just call mine 'the cancer diet.'"

Ignoring Cheryl's attempt at gallows humor, I leaned forward and replied, "You and Marc have obviously made considerable progress with the wedding planning. But how have you been spending the rest of your time? What have you been doing today, for instance?"

"Not much," Cheryl answered as her smile evaporated. "At this point, I can't even seem to focus on my stocks. Maybe that shouldn't come as a big surprise. As every smart investor knows, value only accrues over the long term, which, to put it mildly, is not how I'm currently 'positioned.'"

Yet I could think of another reason for Cheryl's decreasing capacity to concentrate on her investments that additionally explained the ever-increasing number of hours she spent inside her darkened home—it was depression, among the most notorious of terminal illness's many confederates. Depression frequently leads a significant percentage of the terminally-ill to contemplate suicide during the course of their decline.[4]

4. See, e.g., William Breibart, MD, Barry Rosenfeld, PhD, Hayley Pessin, MA, Monique Kaim, PhD, Julie Funesti-Esch, RN, Michele Galietta, MA, Christian J. Nelson, MA, and Robert Brescia, "Depression, Hopelessness, and Desire for Hastened Death in Terminally Ill Patients With Cancer," *Journal of the American Medical Association* 284 (December 13, 2000) 2907–11. As the article's abstract emphasizes: "Desire for hastened death among terminally ill cancer patients is not uncommon. Depression and hopelessness are the strongest predictors of desire for hastened death in this population and provide independent and unique contributions. Interventions addressing depression, hopelessness, and

I always kept that fact in mind when I completed the section of my hospice documentation form reserved for "Plan of Care." A nurse treating a patient beset by a bedsore might, for instance, list a series of interventions: "Turn patient, clean wound, medicate wound, bandage wound." But no similar step-by-step remedy exists for healing patients afflicted with depression. To be sure, anti-depressants, psychotherapy, and even good, old-fashioned handholding each can play a part in loosening depression's grip. That said, however, Psalm 30:6 may still furnish the keenest insight about depression: "Weeping may lodge overnight, but joy may take up residence at morning." Depression can lift, in other words, with all the suddenness it descended; persisting through depression for a little longer can thus spell the difference between night and day.[5] If I were to devise a plan of care to get Cheryl through her depression, it had to include a mechanism for propelling her from one day to the next.

"Cheryl," I asked, "do you and Marc still date?"

She and Marc looked at me dumbfounded. I repeated my question: "Do the two of you still go out on dates?"

"What do you mean?!" she lashed back as her voice rose with anger. "You, of all people, should know how sick I am!"

"I do know, Cheryl," I said, intentionally keeping my voice low and even in counterpoise to hers. "But I also know you're well enough to go out to shop for a wedding dress. I'm merely suggesting that you additionally go out on dates with your fiancé until your 'big day' arrives. I'm not saying you should go out dancing all night—only that you go out each day to someplace the two of you might enjoy.

"Cheryl, you've asked me to assist you with religious services, and I've agreed. But I'm here more basically to help provide you spiritual support, and from the very first, I've seen what raises your spirits most: the chance to share with Marc whatever time you have left remaining. It's in *that* spirit, isn't it, that you've decided to get married to each other? But why limit that time to your wedding? Why confine it to a dark living room? You and Marc pride yourselves on being 'realists.' You know you're going to decline. You just don't know how soon. Why not capitalize on the

---

social support appear to be important aspects of adequate palliative care, particularly, as it relates to desire for hastened death." In the article, patients' "desire for hastened death" refers to physician-assisted suicide.

5. William Styron makes this very point in his book, *Darkness Visible: A Memoir of Madness* (New York: Random House, 1990).

strength you still possess to reap whatever joy it could bring you, starting now, *today*?"

Cheryl stared at me as if she were mulling over a proposed real estate venture. After a long silence, she at last replied, "Point taken." Then, she turned to Marc and said, "You know, Honey, we haven't gone to a movie for a while, particularly to a comedy. Besides, in a movie theater, who will be able to see how the hell I look?"

"It's a date!" Marc said, grinning.

"Don't get home too late!" yelped Helen. "You know I don't like to be alone at night."

Still looking at Marc, Cheryl answered, "Don't worry, Ma. We'll watch the clock."

But I knew that dealing with Cheryl's depression required more than "Movies with Marc." Injecting myself—and the objectives of my plan of care—back into the conversation, I said, "Cheryl, if you're going to keep your spirits up from day to day, then *every* day you need to leverage whatever energy you've got to do something that simply makes you feel good, however briefly. Look, I know you and Marc like to organize and plan. So why not draw up a list of possible pursuits and then categorize them with an eye towards your likely capabilities? Sort them, for example, into those you could perform on the spur of the moment, those you could carry of with advance preparation, and finally, those you would deem doubtful by any measure. Bottom line, Cheryl, stay on the lookout for at least one activity each day that will give you pleasure. What do you say?"

"Well," said Cheryl, "it sure beats sitting around the house waiting to die."

"Great!" I responded, feeling relieved that I had helped Cheryl handle her depression—if only for a day. "When I see you again next week, I'll look forward to hearing about your exploits."

"See you same day and time, Rabbi?" Marc asked, pulling out his PDA.

"Sure thing. But obviously, if you need to see me sooner, just call the office and have them page me." Marc smiled broadly as he shook my hand. I got my things together and stepped outside. The rain had stopped, and any remaining overcast had cleared.

I drove back to Cheryl's a week later with high hopes of hearing word of her improvement. They were short-lived, however. For the first time, Cheryl didn't open the door—Marc did, his face drawn and pallid.

Without a word, he led me to Cheryl and Helen in the living room where I was greeted by another first: the shades had been raised, and sunlight poured through the panes of the large bay window. But whenever a beam of light fell on Cheryl, it cast a warning beacon on her complexion, illumining pancreatic cancer's telltale yellow tint signaling the deadly menace's spread beneath.

"Thanks for coming, Rabbi. But the visit is going to have to be short today. Cheryl's really not feeling well."

"*That's* an understatement!" Helen barked. "She's in a lot of pain."

"OK, Cheryl," I said, "rate your pain level for me."

"It's about a '5.'"

From her first day on hospice, Cheryl would have heard about effective pain management, which is not merely hospice's area of specialization, but its very reason for existence. Good hospice care depends on giving patients and their caregivers good hospice education, which not infrequently involves providing repeated *re*-education. Cheryl's reported pain level meant I needed to review with her the basics of pain control.

"You probably already know, Cheryl, that once the pain level reaches a '3' or a '4', it's time for you to call the hospice office so they can advise you how to lower it as speedily and as safely as possible."

"Yeah, I know. Billie, the nurse, has told me that before, but I figure I'll wait until she gets here to take care of it."

"Cheryl," I countered, "staying 'ahead of the pain' is important for hospice patients. Think about when you've had a headache. Sometimes, you've probably said to yourself, 'It's not that bad; I can tolerate the pain a while longer before I do something about it.' But then something distracts or delays you, and more time passes before you finally get around to taking something to relieve the headache. Meanwhile, the pain has worsened. By the time you finally *do* take a pain reliever, the medication takes just that much longer to begin to work. The same thing is true for pain medication for cancer patients—except that your pain is typically much more severe than the kind generally associated with some run-of-the-mill headache."

I didn't wait for any rejoinder from Cheryl. Billie had probably already left her the appropriate medication as well as instructions for taking it. But however much I might want to expedite matters, dispensing medication lay beyond my legitimate scope of practice, and I had no authority to direct Cheryl to up her dosage.

"Cheryl, with your permission, I'd like to call the office and tell them what you just told me."

"Go ahead. The phone's in the kitchen."

I excused myself and called the office. By chance, Carmen, our hospice's Patient Care Administrator—its "Nurse of Nurses"—answered the phone. When I repeated Cheryl's pain level to her, she asked to speak to Cheryl personally; she wanted to make sure that Cheryl understood not only the instructions for increasing her medication's amount, but also *the need* for increasing it.

As soon as Cheryl had left the living room to take Carmen's call in the kitchen, Marc began to speak in a voice that, though hushed, still rasped with exasperation. "Look, Rabbi, your staff has had this discussion with Cheryl more than once. But none of you really seems to grasp the reason for her resistance to the drugs. Although she may have accepted her physical deterioration, she regards any potential sign of her weakening psychologically as totally unacceptable. That's why she has turned down cancer support groups and individual psychotherapy—and why she refuses to take her pain medication. Cheryl genuinely believes that she can withstand her pain by relying on the same strength of will, the same sheer grit, that has sustained her since childhood."

"I can appreciate your frustration, Marc," I replied. "I think your explanation of Cheryl's resistance to the painkillers makes a good deal of sense, especially in light of her personal history. Tell you what. Let's see what she has to say when she gets off the phone and pick up the discussion from there."

About ten minutes later, Cheryl re-entered the living room. Helen looked up and asked, "Well, what did they have to tell you?"

"Same old, same old: increase the dosage and, if need be, the frequency of the meds. But like I told them—this level of pain is bearable. I mean, I want to save the drugs for when I really need them!"

"Cheryl," I responded, "the choice whether or not to take the meds ultimately remains yours. But from the first time I met you, you've struck me as somebody who can't stand any sugarcoating of the truth. So let me give it to you straight: despite your best efforts to 'beat the pain' by willpower alone, the pain will eventually nevertheless *always beat you*—just like it does everybody else. The longer you delay taking your meds when you're in pain, the more you've wasted what little time you've got left. Taking the meds is no sign of being weak: it's a sign of being smart."

Whether overcome by the power of my logic, or more plausibly, by the potency of her pain, Cheryl capitulated. "OK, OK, already. You were right that going out with Marc would make me feel better, and maybe you're right about this, too. Ma, will you go into the kitchen and get me a glass of water so I can go ahead and take the damn pills?"

As Helen returned with the pills and a glass of water, I wanted to reinforce Cheryl's decision by combining my knowledge of pain management with what I knew of her. "I realize from our past talks that being in control means a great deal to you and Marc. There's nothing wrong about that; you've both made successes of your lives precisely because you've managed to exert control in facing various complex challenges. But this illness means that more and more frequently, you'll have less and less control over a whole host of things. With hospice's help, pain doesn't have to be one of them. Keeping 'ahead of your pain' means maintaining control over it."

"Enough—I heard you," said Cheryl as she took the glass of water from Helen and swallowed the pain pills. "I know I'm going downhill, and part of me doesn't want to face up to it. As much as I tell myself that I'm prepared for all this, maybe, in the end, I'm really not. But as I've said before, I think I succeeded as an investor, because I always made fact-based decisions. If I'm going to deal with my pain more successfully, I better start facing facts a whole lot more realistically."

"That's my Cheryl!" Marc exulted as he put his arm around her.

Just then, the doorbell rang. Marc got up, went to answer it, and came back with Billie.

"Hi, everybody," she said. "How are things going today?"

"Tell you what, Billie," I answered, "I've got to run to my next appointment. I'll let everybody else fill you in." Of course, Billie and I knew that we, like every other member of the hospice team, would update one another at day's end with voicemail messages assessing Cheryl's condition (as well as Marc's and Helen's) from our respective discipline's perspective. Indeed, when I checked my voicemail late that afternoon and listened to Billie's subsequent summary of her nurse's visit, it only confirmed what I had earlier surmised: "Cheryl's in much worse shape than when I last saw her a few days ago. I only hope she can hang on long enough for her and Marc to have their wedding."

The next voicemail in the queue gave Billie's added urgency. It came from Jeff, the social worker assigned to Cheryl's case: "Hi, Michael. I called the house today to schedule a visit tomorrow. I ended up speaking with Marc. He says he's got his hands full making sure that Helen's financial future is secure after Cheryl dies. But Cheryl herself has told me that Marc completed all the steps necessary to provide for Helen's basic welfare weeks ago. Marc's continuing focus on her mother instead of her upsets her enormously. It dredges up all the resentment Cheryl has harbored since childhood toward Helen and Helen's neediness. And truthfully, Michael, who can argue with Cheryl's resentfulness or, for that matter, with her renewed sense of abandonment? If she can't get Marc's full attention and total commitment now, when can she ever hope to?"

I knew I had to act quickly if I were to be of any help. I immediately paged Billie and Jeff to find out when they had slotted their next visits with Cheryl; I wanted to avoid scheduling three hospice appointments on the same day. I found a day later that week free of any hospice calls whatsoever, and I phoned Marc to ask whether I might come by earlier than arranged. Not entirely fallaciously, I explained that some pressing matters had arisen that had complicated my schedule. "Would you mind," I asked, "if I came by the day after tomorrow?"

"Not at all, Rabbi," he replied, "we're always glad to see you."

When I arrived at the condo, Marc again met me at the door. No longer a walking ad straight out of a man's fashion magazine, he stood before me rumpled, red-eyed, and unshaven. "Excuse my appearance," he began, "but I've been up all night with Cheryl. She's upstairs sleeping—finally. She can't keep anything at all down now, and she's started to have to take increasingly more of the morphine, which leaves her less and less lucid. On top of everything else, I've still got some loose ends I need to tie up concerning Helen's finances. Thank God, I've got her out of the house running some errands."

I asked Marc if we might go up to Cheryl's room to speak. I thought I had a better chance to make my case—*Cheryl's case*—by her bedside. When we reached the bedroom, Cheryl still lay fast asleep, and I could see for myself how much she had deteriorated in the mere two days since my last visit.

"Marc," I said taking a seat, "from now on, Cheryl's liable to have more days like this one. So let me put a question to you: although the financial arrangements you've made for Helen may fall short of your ideal efforts, do you think they're adequate overall?"

"I'm not sure, Rabbi. It always feel as though there's something more I could or should be doing."

"Marc, by your simply *being* with Cheryl now, you're *doing* the most important thing of all, because it's quite literally something death-defying: affirming the value of her life, and of yours, and of your love for one another. Remember what Cheryl answered me when I first asked why you two wanted to get married regardless of her illness? She said she wanted 'to experience the joy of a wedding' and any subsequent time, however long or short, she might have to spend with you—not *despite of* but *on account of* what you both knew awaited her. Why not go ahead then, Marc, and get married as soon as possible, maybe even in the next day or two? What's the worst that can happen? You'll simply have that much more time to spend together afterwards as an 'old married couple.'"

Marc sucked in a deep breath and held it for a few moments before letting it out again. "I'll start to get things rolling, Rabbi." He was about to say something else when the front door opened. "Marc, it's Helen! I'm home! I could use a hand with these shopping bags!"

Marc and I arose and went back downstairs. When Helen saw me, she gasped, "My God, has Cheryl died?!"

"You must have forgotten, Helen," Marc said gently. "I mentioned to you that Rabbi Goldberg would be coming by this afternoon due to some changes in his schedule."

Still rattled, Helen began to cry. "Did you see, Rabbi, how bad my poor Cheryl looks? How long do you think she has?"

"I don't have the answer to that question, Helen. Nobody does, I think, except God: just as only God knows the exact moment we're going to enter this world, so too, God alone knows the split second we're going to depart it. As a result, I believe in living life with plans that are more pliable than rigid, especially when life is at its edges, as Cheryl's is right now. Let's therefore tentatively agree that I'll return the day after tomorrow—*with* the proviso that if you need to see me sooner, you'll have the office page me."

Marc and Helen nodded, and both appeared more at ease. Meanwhile, Cheryl had remained asleep during the entire visit.

Two days later, as I pulled up in front of another patient's home to begin a scheduled visit, I got a page displaying Billie's phone number, followed by "911," the code for "Urgent!"

"Listen, Michael," Billie said, after I called her back, "I'm over at Cheryl's now. I know you're supposed to come out here later this afternoon, but I think she may be in the process of actively dying. Of course, I don't know how long that might take. But I do know that if she and Marc are going to get married, they need to do it today! Marc is trying to reach his own rabbi, but so far, no luck. It's the rabbi's day off, and his office hasn't been able to locate him. How soon can you get over here? One way or another, whether for a wedding or for a bereavement, they could use a rabbi ASAP."

"I'll get there as soon as I can, Billie, but unfortunately, I've just arrived at Bob Livingston's house to keep an appointment with him." Because Bob was a patient whom Billie and I both saw, she knew he lived miles away from Cheryl. "Billie," I continued, "tell Marc I'll get there as quickly as possible, but meantime, let's hope somebody gets hold of Rabbi Slatkin."

I went inside to talk with Bob. Luckily, since our last appointment, no new issues had developed and no outstanding ones remained, and consequently, the visit went routinely—i.e., swiftly—thus freeing me to leave for Cheryl's earlier than anticipated. When I got back in my car, I called Marc on my cell phone. "Marc, this is Rabbi Goldberg. I'm heading over now. What's going on at your end?"

"Thank God, we finally reached Rabbi Slatkin. He ought to be here any minute. Meanwhile, Billie and a couple of the hospice aides are already here, and they've done so much more than lower Cheryl's pain—they've taken charge of the set-up for the ceremony: arranging flowers, putting out refreshments, and, best of all, helping Cheryl with her wedding gown. They might as well be bridesmaids!"

"That's grand that things are going so well," I said, genuinely pleased. "Even though you don't seem to need me for the *chuppah*,[6] would you mind if I stopped by for the *simchah*?"[7]

"By all means, Rabbi! Drop by anytime."

As events unfolded, Marc's open-ended invitation proved fortuitous. An accident several miles up the freeway turned a typically thirty-minute cruise into a two-hour crawl. When I at last set foot in Cheryl's condo, Helen caught sight of me and proceeded to report that I had missed the wedding as well as Rabbi Slatkin, who, she informed me, had left long ago.

6. Hebrew for "wedding ceremony."

7. Hebrew for "joyous occasion"—in this case, the celebration following the ceremony *per se*.

Many of the newlyweds' friends and family nonetheless remained—along with plenty to eat and drink, a traditional hallmark of any Jewish wedding, regardless of the circumstances. The sofa had been moved to the center of the living room, and on it sat Cheryl and Marc having their pictures taken. As visibly happy as they appeared, I couldn't help but notice a difference between their picture-taking session and those of other just-married couples: in between each snapshot, a hospice aide affixed another safety-pin to Cheryl's gown to better drape it over her wasted torso.

I made my way through the other guests to offer my congratulations. "*Mazal Tov!*" I cried out. "I can't tell you how happy I am for the two of you! I'm just sorry I wasn't able to make it in time for the ceremony."

Whether trying to conserve Cheryl's strength, or simply unable to contain his own excitement, Marc spoke up and recounted the day's sequence of events. "This morning, after another pretty bad night, Cheryl insisted on our getting married today, no 'ifs,' 'ands,' or 'buts.' So I tried to get in touch with Rabbi Slatkin. Next, I made a bunch of calls to family and friends to pick up food and flowers. By then, I had to phone your office, because *mittendrinnen*,[8] Cheryl's pain level had shot up to '7.' When I told them that Cheryl wanted to hold the wedding today come hell or high water ... well, you've already heard about the exceptional work your hospice staff did after that."

Suddenly, I noticed Cheryl wincing. "Cheryl," I asked, "do you need another dose of your meds?"

With the pain progressing and the ceremony now concluded, she put up no resistance. "Yeah, I suppose so. Anyway, if other people around here are taking shots of booze to help them get a little happy, then I'll have a shot of morphine as my own little pick-me-up!" Soon after her morphine was administered, Cheryl's pain subsided, and when I left half-an-hour later, she was still sitting on the sofa holding court the same as any other brand new bride.

And yet, the newlyweds' bliss offered them no immunity from Cheryl's cancer's onslaught. Within forty-eight hours of the wedding, I received an emergency call from Carmen. "Michael, I just heard from Billie. She's at Cheryl's, and she says Cheryl is really declining rapidly now. The wedding may have wrung Cheryl's last drop of strength out of her. You should get over there as quickly as you can."

---

8. Yiddish for "in the midst of everything."

I thanked Carmen, hung up, and dialed Cheryl's. Helen answered. Her voice, always fearful, sounded absolutely terrified. "Rabbi, thank God, it's you. Come over right away! I think we're about to lose Cheryl. Marc's been sitting upstairs in bed with her for hours. I don't know what to do. Please come over!" I let her know I was on my way.

For once, neither traffic nor parking posed a problem. Marc answered the door. The terror on his face matched that in Helen's voice. "Thanks for coming, Rabbi. Cheryl is upstairs sleeping; ever since the wedding, that's what she's spent most of the time doing."

We went up to the bedroom where Cheryl appeared to lie deep asleep. Helen sat in a chair drawn up beside her. I knew my hospice always left behind an information booklet for families and other caregivers following our first patient visit. I looked directly into Marc's eyes and recited one of its passages verbatim: "The nearer a patient's approach to death, the less time generally spent awake." Turning his gaze away from mine and lowering his voice, Marc replied, "Yes, they've told us that more than once. Helen and I have agreed to take shifts with Cheryl so that when the end comes, she won't be alone."

"Loving Cheryl the way you two do, I can't imagine your wanting to be anyplace *but* by her side," I said, speaking softly. "As you stay with her, though, try to keep your expectations of yourselves—and of Cheryl—realistic, just the way she herself would want it.

"Here's what I mean. Sometimes we cast an aura of 'romanticism' around death and dying. Our culture is replete, for instance, with stories in which family and friends hold round-the-clock death-bed vigils, waiting for the one approaching death to utter some concluding words chock-full of meaning that ultimately speak louder than death itself. In those stories, as ancient as the Bible's and as current as Hollywood's latest blockbuster, the dying draw one last breath and convey some 'immortal truth of life' along with their undying love for those gathered round the bedside.

"But Marc and Helen, those deathbed scenes, for all their poignancy, fail to portray the way most people pass away. By and large, the dying simply *die*; after having lost consciousness, they generally don't regain it, much less some capacity to speak any 'final words of wisdom.' Cheryl may never say another word to you again, whether or not you maintain a constant deathwatch by her bed. Consequently, in the end, however much or little time you sit with her from this point forward matters far less than all the time you've spent with her up to now. Solace lies in recalling all *that* time, because that's where you'll be put most in mind not only of all those instances of your love for Cheryl, but equally important, of hers for you."

Tears streamed down Helen's face, and Marc began to sob.

I suggested we take each other's hands—Cheryl's included—and recite the *Shema*,[9] the words traditionally said at or near the time of a Jew's death. Afterwards, all of us sat silently for several moments, our eyes fixed on Cheryl's face, each deep in his or her own thoughts. I looked down at my watch and saw I needed to leave to go to another patient's home. "Marc and Helen," I said as I excused myself, "try to get some more sleep; call me if you need me." I got up, went downstairs, and let myself out.

The next morning as I was about to start out on my route, the phone rang. "Michael, this is Carmen. I thought you should know. Cheryl died last night."

Although the news came as no surprise, it still stunned me. While I would hardly have described Cheryl as the warmest person I had ever met, I suddenly missed her fire, and for the rest of the morning, I remained virtually frozen. I found myself unable to take even the smallest steps toward performing the one last act of care I had promised her: presiding at her funeral.

Eventually, I phoned the condo, composing myself as best I could. Marc answered. I offered my condolences and reaffirmed my commitment to officiate at Cheryl's burial. I could hear the sense of relief in Marc's voice, now that he had one less item requiring his attention. He thanked me, and then he broke down. "Helen and I tried to follow the advice you gave us yesterday, Rabbi, but we couldn't quite pull ourselves away from Cheryl's bedside altogether. Instead, I carried two easy chairs upstairs from the living room and placed them by her bed so we could stay there with her, catching catnaps as best we could. Around three o'clock this morning, I must have nodded off. After a little while, Helen got up to go to the bathroom right off Cheryl's bedroom. When Helen returned, a minute or two later at most, Cheryl was gone. Who knows? Maybe it was mere coincidence. Or maybe it was simply Cheryl being 'Cheryl', determined to die the same way she lived—by nobody's lights but her own."

Two days earlier, I had offered counsel at Cheryl's deathbed. Two days preceding that, I had offered congratulations at her wedding. And in just two days hence, I would offer comfort at her funeral.

9. The opening word, in Hebrew, of Deut 6:3: "Hear [O Israel] . . ."

Cheryl's Torso

Such a chronology of events might lead some to question the point of Marc and Cheryl getting married in the first place. But such a question misses "the point" entirely. Certain things have no point beyond themselves. Rather, they are ends in themselves, to be valued as good for their own sake and on their own account. Life is one such thing, love another, and joy a third. Who knew that better than Cheryl and Marc? And what story better attests to that than theirs?

8

Thad's Heart

STORIES HAVE SO FAR comprised this book, and so, not surprisingly, a story will conclude it, too—but of a different sort. The preceding ones have portrayed me as my patients' chaplain, they and I strangers whose paths might have never crossed except for the unexpected thump they heard one day resounding from death's door. This closing narrative, however, places me not as a chaplain beside some sick stranger's bed, but as a friend alongside a friend who ended up more than friend, and who started out as teacher directing me to stories in the first place. So, I cannot tell some of his story apart from telling some of mine, as against both our wills, he edged ever closer to death's doorstep.

❀   ❀   ❀

"'Scuse me, fellas, but I hafta take a pee," said the man to his decades-younger lunch companions at the dinky local taqueria, his coarse language so jarringly at odds with his typically genteel Southern manner. The scene could have served as a snapshot of his long career as he sat with students roundabout him—three current ones from Southern California and the other, myself, from twenty years before, down visiting from the state's other end, to which I had returned. Though in his seventies now and slightly stooped when he got up, Thad still stood lanky, over six feet tall, his neatly-groomed silver beard and head of hair encircling his face's high-boned, ruddy cheeks, its center a perpetually reddish nose, symptomatic not, as some might have supposed, of an alcoholic—despite his partiality to a Beefeater Martini every afternoon at five—but of another sickness altogether, one known by its inevitable result: Congestive Heart Failure. Like the other medications that he took, Thad's diuretics, responsible for his frequent need to urinate, could only slow but by no means stop the disease's relentless course.[1]

But twenty years earlier in a doctoral seminar of his, as I sat over books on philosophy and religion instead of plates of tacos and burritos, neither of us could have foreseen such an outcome to his life—or the impact it would have on mine. In fact, only a few months before enrolling in that seminar and in the larger program of which it was a part, I could scarcely have imagined myself in such a setting in any case—surrounded by Christians, most preparing for ministry, some, like myself, for the academy, but all with a religious tradition distinctly different from my own.

Fresh out of rabbinical school, I had come to Thad, because, frankly, I had no place else to turn to pursue the career I had pictured for myself. I had not entered seminary to emerge a rabbi in a synagogue, much less a chaplain in a hospital, hospice, or nursing home. Rather, I had gone to seminary as a stepping stone on a professional path leading, in my mind's eye, to a world entirely removed from those, that of a secular university. Within those ivied walls, I would write and teach about the philosophy of religion in all its subtleties. Because, like most American Jews, I had grown up with little grounding in such traditional Jewish texts as the Bible, the Talmud, and the classical legal codes, rabbinical school consequently seemed a necessary, if inconvenient, stop en route to realizing my academic ambitions.

But the possibility of seminary as a stopover on some spiritual quest never so much as flitted through my brain, the piece of myself I prized back then more than any other. On the days when I wasn't an out-and-out atheist, I was no conventional agnostic, but instead, more grandiloquently, an "*ignostic*": God's existence, even if properly defined and proved, made no more difference to my daily life than did Bigfoot's. Happily, the Deity's existence didn't seem to make much difference day-to-day to my seminary, either. I used to joke that, for the sake of truth in advertising, the place should cease peddling itself as a "theological seminary" in favor of a more accurate rebranding—that of a "theological *cemetery*," its motto reading: "The only good God is a dead God." The five-year ordination track, virtually empty of electives, required but one course in "theology," an overview of Jewish prayer. While the class devoted itself to studying

1. Some readers, no doubt, will be able to uncover Thad's identity despite my changing his name. Yet change it I have, for like every other person in this book (and in this chapter), respect for him and his survivors requires nothing less.

various prayers' historical contexts and historic changes, it studiously avoided discussing those prayers' own object of devotion: God.

Yet the more my classes evaded questions about God, the more I found myself strangely preoccupied by them: did belief in God, for instance, rest on "Revelation"—or could it be derived from "Reason"?; did "Morality" similarly depend on divine decree—or might it be inferred from some independent form of "Rationality"?; and, perhaps most perplexing of all to me, did "Religion" function as *the* font of "Truth" for human life—or merely as one well of "Meaning" among others? Such quandaries, I knew, had bedeviled philosophers and theologians for centuries, and as I neared the end of seminary, I found that somehow despite myself, these mind-baffling puzzles had now cast their spell on me. As a result, I started casting around for a doctoral program that might hold the key—some analytic method!—to set me free of the conceptual conundrums that so possessed me. And yet, of the doctoral programs I explored, the Jewish ones expressed no particular interest in addressing abstract questions regarding God, the Christian ones exhibited no great enthusiasm concerning me, and the secular ones showed no sympathy for "the philosophy of religion" whatsoever.

Eventually, however, a former teacher, himself a rabbi, but whose own institution awarded no doctorate, directed me to Thad, whom he had met at a symposium that included faculty from the ecumenical graduate consortium where Thad taught Christian ethics. I subsequently phoned Thad, and in that bi-coastal conversation, I circumspectly sketched my academic field of inquiry, my preference for a philosophical approach to it, and finally, and still more guardedly, my own religious background. None of the three put Thad off: on the contrary, he welcomed all of them together.

My work with Thad began when I signed up for a seminar he led on justifying our convictions. These are our core beliefs—be they religious, moral, political, or some other kind—that we, as communities and as individuals, embody in our key practices and thus ultimately play out *in life*. In the seminar, however, such notions played around only inside my head. To me, the whole enterprise of dissecting diverse authors' disparate views appeared an exercise akin to cracking a crossword in the *New York Times*, or, in other words, an activity requiring nimble wits, but nothing more—a sentiment I hastened to verbalize midway through the course. In rabbinical school, my remark would have evoked, at best, a stern stare from the course instructor and, at worst, a sterner call for my withdrawal from the ordination track at once. But Thad replied to what I'd said without any disapproving glare or withering riposte, saying soft-spokenly and simply, "Well, Michael, I need to think about that a while." Although he obviously cared about the seminar and its subject matter, he cared more about me, and not only me, but also the other students in the class. He cared about the effect his response would have on *all* our lives—his own included. To him, the true justifiability of a conviction lay not in the validity of an argument made within a book, but in the justifiability of a life lived in the world outside it.

For Thad, one life, more than any other, displayed the justifiability of a life lived—Jesus'—and not only in the world of Jesus' own time, but for all time thereafter. Thad liked to call himself a "small 'b' baptist" (in contrast to the bombastic, big 'B' Southern Baptists to whom so many Americans have become accustomed—and allergic), aligning himself with a variety of Anabaptists, medieval as well as modern, committed to the practice of non-violence based on their convictions about following Jesus' way. For "small 'b' baptists" such as these, Jesus in both word and deed had repudiated violence at every step—from his teaching on the Mount[2] to his arrest in Gethsemane[3] to his crucifixion at Calvary.[4] From first to last, he had rejected retaliation against enemies as a way of making peace, even though it had cost him dearly.

For Thad, too, Jesus' way had proved a costly one. During the American escalation in Vietnam, he held a teaching post at an ostensibly Christian institution. Using that platform to full effect, Thad publicly spoke out against any further expansion of the war, wrote articles echoing that opposition, and, in an act that proved too much for the school's administration, joined with students voicing their own dissent. Taking a page from some holy writ other than the Gospels, the administrators chose to fire the peacemaker rather than to bless him. A short time earlier, another putatively "Christian" seminary had also terminated Thad, his

2. See, e.g., Matt 5:39, "If anyone slaps you on the right cheek, turn and offer him the other also," and Luke 6:29, "If anyone hits you on the cheek, offer the other also." (Revised English Bible; I use this version due, in part, to Thad's own preference for it.)

3. See, e.g., Matt 26:52: "Put up your sword. All who take the sword die by the sword" (REB).

4. See, e.g., Luke 23:34: "Father, forgive them; they do not know what they are doing" (REB).

tenure notwithstanding, for raising money to help students get to Selma, where, alongside Dr. King, they would practice Christian non-violence in hopes of ending segregation. Forever wounded by the whole affair, Thad once grimly observed to me, "All tenure means is that they have to lynch you legal." But for Thad, it seemed, following in Jesus' steps meant expecting nothing less; after all, Jesus' own career had been abruptly interrupted, complete with a full array of legal trappings.

For my part, though, I could not begin to fathom how Thad or *anyone* could take such risks based on some religion's teaching. To my mind, the significance of religious teaching, whatever its alleged origin, rested not in its truth, but in its utility;[5] high-flown palaver regarding "God's Transcendence" mattered far less to me than down-to-earth discourse concerning Jews' group solidarity and its implications for their survival. When the seminar concluded its last session three months later, I lingered until the room had emptied out, save for Thad and me. I wanted to speak to him by himself, free from the cross-talk, in every sense, of the other students, for what I had to say to Thad might well have rivaled, indeed outstripped, in its apparent *chutzpah* my comment about convictions and crosswords made several weeks before. During that period, however, one far-reaching change had been set in motion—not that I had begun valuing my own views any less, but that I had started esteeming Thad far more.

"You know," I said to him as he slid the last of his papers back inside his briefcase, "I'm not at all sure that if, for instance, the Exodus from Egypt had never happened, Judaism would necessarily be undermined. I mean, if two guys named Nate and Al had made up the whole story hundreds of years later while sitting around a campfire in the Galilee one night to amuse themselves because they had nothing else to do, I don't think it would make one iota of difference to how Jews think or act. For us, unlike for Christians, our practices have always taken precedence over our beliefs."

As before, Thad responded without any hint of rancor. He took some moments to ponder what I'd said, still more to mull over his reply, finally answering in his characteristically low and gentle voice, "I'm not so sure, Michael. I can't speak for Jews and Judaism, of course. But for Christians, it would make all the difference in the world if there were no resurrec-

---

5. My views had their source in such "Jewish" thinkers as, for instance, Spinoza, Durkheim, and Mordecai Kaplan as well as in such non-Jewish ones as Dewey and William James.

tion. It's the heart of the good news of God's undying love for us, given us no matter what. Without the resurrection, violence would always trump forgiveness and peace-making, its partner, and Christian hopes of life beyond the one we have here on earth, however sincerely cherished, would simply go unjustified. If the resurrection never happened, Michael, Jesus' story would be *just* a story."

For me, an initially God-indifferent Jew, Jesus' story became more than "just a story" through the way Thad continually enacted it in the story that unfolded between the two of us. Long after I had finished my formal training with him and received my doctoral degree—along with an (Exodus-dependent!) degree of belief in God besides[6]—Thad served as my steadfastly open-minded mentor, open-hearted confidant, and even, when the need arose, open-handed benefactor. Whether in his office, at his home, or over the phone long-distance, he truly ministered to me, never trying to convert me to Christianity, but always listening patiently to my predicaments, regardless of their having stemmed from my conviction or sprung from my impulsiveness. Then, ever-sensitive to the possibility of shaming me, that soothing baritone of his would delicately propose an alternative approach that might work better. Invariably, he would close our conversation saying, "Lovely to speak with you, Michael. I love you, and so does God." Thanks to Thad, I gained the skills not only to become an academic who could delve into the great religious stories of the past but, in due time, a chaplain who could sound out the humbler ones of patients struggling with whatever future they had left.

The years passed by. I moved all around the country while Thad packed up but once, traveling to join his wife, Kath, in Southern California at the seminary that had offered her a professorship and him a distinguished-scholar-in-residence position. Suddenly one morning, Thad, by now in his late-sixties, woke up with trouble breathing. Kath drove him to his primary physician, and a battery of diagnostic tests revealed Congestive Heart Failure as the underlying complaint, the same malady which had killed both his parents before either's reaching seventy. A cardiologist, Dr. MacManus, consequently took over, managing Thad's care through interventions ranging from drugs to diet—although, as Thad admitted to me

---

6. Cf., e.g., my *Jews and Christians, Getting Our Stories Straight: The Exodus and the Passion-Resurrection* (Eugene, OR: Wipf & Stock, 2001), and *Why Should Jews Survive?: Looking Past the Holocaust Toward a Jewish Future* (New York: Oxford University Press, 1996).

early on, he didn't always follow doctor's orders, especially the one nixing his late-afternoon martini.

But despite all the physical and medical changes in his life, Thad's commitment to the Christian life remained ostensibly as firm as ever. When the small, foundering church to which he and Kath belonged asked him to become its part-time pastor for a year as it tried to right itself, Thad consented rather than beg off due to either age or illness. Nor did he rely on either as rationales for reducing his teaching load or retiring from teaching altogether. Finally, he refused to let his advanced years or his advancing ailment impede his scholarly publication: he revised a previous book, wrote two new ones, and started work on the third and final volume of his "small 'b' baptist" understanding of the Christian life, a project that by then had engaged him for close to twenty years.

And yet, however much Thad kept going, so, also, did his disease, its course not merely chronic but degenerative. To keep a step ahead, Dr. MacManus had to resort to an ever-expanding spate of drugs. But for all his skill and care in extending Thad's life well beyond the years allotted it by a typical prognosis, no physician's art could have anticipated the would-be turning point of Thad's decline. With Kath away giving lectures overseas, Thad went out for dinner at a local restaurant, where he ate contaminated seafood, returning home so sick from diarrhea that he landed in a nearby hospital's ICU, his potassium levels having plummeted to almost fatal levels. Although Thad recovered from the episode, Dr. MacManus realized its import. He advised that Thad have a defibrillator implant, and Thad agreed.

Some six months later, the device went off. Kath, at home furiously trying to scribble down all Thad's meds before driving him to the hospital herself, frantically rang Dr. MacManus, who instructed her to call "911" instead. The ambulance took Thad to the emergency room, where he got pumped full of diuretics. He returned home three days after that, even weaker than before. During his recuperation, I phoned him from my home in Northern California. He told me the defibrillator had fired half a dozen times in thirty minutes. When I asked him what it felt like, he replied by asking me a question of his own: "Have you ever stuck your finger in a 120-volt electric socket?"

From that time forward, Thad grew increasingly anxious about the defibrillator's going off again and jolting his whole system. To calm him down, Dr. MacManus prescribed the anti-anxiety medication, Xanax.

Thad popped the pills like Pez. A single dose of Xanax, intended to last four hours, often wore off on Thad after a mere two or three, leaving his anxiety unabated, if not amplified, as his damaged heart beat in tandem with his fretful one.[7]

Trying to reassert control over his disease and distress together, Thad began what Kath dubbed "his grand tour of manliness." He traded his little red two-seater for a large silver pick-up truck and explained to Kath his raison d'être: "I want to make sure I have momentum on my side to survive any accidents." (To me, he explained his reasoning for carrying a pickle jar onboard: "To prevent any accidents on account of the diuretics.") That summer, he drove off in his new vehicle to his boyhood home in the sultry South—where he promptly collapsed, thus requiring complex arrangements to stabilize him and fly him back to California. Then, virtually in spite of all that had so recently transpired, he trekked off to Santa Fe, its heat and high altitude acutely testing both his heart and lungs once more. Finally, he headed out on horseback for a fishing trip in the Sierras. Whether taken as feats of defiance or as acts of denial, Thad's exploits represented the actions of a man hardly reconciled to dying. But precisely what kind of man? For years, Thad had spoken of God's promising Jesus' followers the power to surmount both suffering and death. Jesus, however, had found the strength to face his fears of dying by praying in a garden—not trout-fishing in the High Sierra.

The final time I saw Thad came by way of one last dinner with him and Kath at the home where I had eaten at their table so many times before. Usually, Thad said grace, but that evening, he asked me to lead it. Whatever I knew about real prayer, rather than the lip service recited rotely in conformity with the dictates of some divinity, dogma, or denomination, I had learned from him. Small wonder, therefore, that in this book's earlier story about "Sally," the hospital patient who had wanted me to pray for her "in Jesus' name," I had turned to Thad for guidance. True prayer, he taught me, took one's whole being—one's head, one's heart, one's *gut*. That night at supper, a prayer poured out of me more gut-wrenching than any I had ever uttered. As Thad had been for me a model of faith in his life, I desperately wanted him to be one in his dying also.[8]

7. This phenomenon, known as "rebound effect," is common to the group of drugs classified as "benzodiazepines," Xanax among them.

8 And, as it turns out, a particular paradigm of Christian faith, at that—namely, the embodiment of the Jesus who simply submits to God's will rather than the one who

"Dear God," I started, "we thank you for this time and meal. But Lord, we recall another time in a garden long ago when, in response to that meal's main course, your beloved son, Jesus, prayed to you, his father, saying, 'If it is possible, let this cup pass by me,' afterwards, however, adding, 'Nevertheless, not according to my will, but yours.'[9] Please, God, let this cup pass by our beloved Thad. But if such is not your will, we pray that you help Thad stay Jesus' faithful follower—like him, faithful to your will." "Amen," said Kath. Thad, though, sat there in stony silence—no "Amen," not even a perfunctory "Thank you, Michael." However slightly unfamiliar the man at lunch had seemed several months ago, the man at dinner now appeared largely unrecognizable.

Although Thad himself may have changed, the symptoms of his decline had not. A short while after our meal together, Thad experienced renewed difficulty breathing. Once again, Dr. MacManus sent him to the hospital to empty the fluid from his lungs; once again, nearly all his potassium got drained out as well; once again, his defibrillator repeatedly went off. The hospital staff told Kath, already at wit's end, he wouldn't live out the night.

Somehow, though, he did—but only barely, without any prospect of his fragile health recovering substantially. A few days following Thad's hospital discharge, Kath contacted his two grown sons by his prior marriage, his psychotherapist, her own spiritual director, and me to collect our thoughts—and hers—about disabling the defibrillator. All of us agreed the device should be disarmed. But when Kath, laying out her heart to Thad, said that since the defibrillator was making both their lives so miserable, the best option might be to turn it off, *he* went off, exploding, "People are miserable in Bosnia, too!" The issue was never discussed between the two of them again. To make sure nobody else thereafter discussed his illness, Thad forbade Kath from divulging to anyone at their seminary just how sick he was.

But while Thad had forbidden Kath from speaking to anyone about the graveness of his condition, he had never prohibited *me* from doing so. Thus when, despite his rapidly deteriorating health, Thad somehow managed to complete the third and final volume of his theological magnum opus, two decades in the making, I phoned back east to his publisher's

---

agonizes on account of it; see, e.g., Matt 27:46 and Mark 15:34, where Jesus, during his crucifixion, cries out, "My God, my God, why have you forsaken me?"

9. Cf. Matt 26:39.

editor-in-chief, informed him of the situation, and asked if an advance copy of the volume, Thad's last in every way, might be sent to him so that he could see it—*touch it!*—before he died. With that sort of deadline looming, the likes of which the publishing house had never run up against before, the editor pledged to use every resource at his command to get a copy of the book into Thad's hands in time.

Soon after, Thad once more found himself in bed gasping desperately for air. He called Dr. MacManus, who, reading from the same script he had followed twice before, recommended a return to the hospital's emergency room. When Thad responded he didn't want to go back there, Dr. MacManus said that such a decision would bring about Thad's death. Thad, worn out, told the cardiologist to come over to the house, shut the defibrillator down, and set him up on hospice.

In the two succeeding weeks, the hospice nurses told Kath they were mystified by Thad's wherewithal to keep on living even as he kept weakening with each passing day. The couple's Hispanic housekeeper, Olivia, whom they had employed for years, a woman of simple education and simple faith, but scarcely simple-minded, prayed by Thad's bedside as he lay sleeping. She prayed that he, like Jesus, trust his soul to God, allow himself to die, and let go of this earthly life for an eternal one.

But Thad still somehow continued to cling to whatever bit of this world's life he still had in him, thus accentuating the apparent theological paradox all the more. If he truly held the resurrection at the core of his convictions, as he had told me in that seminar years before, then why did he display no sense of peace, acceptance, or just sheer resignation as he approached his death?

Meanwhile, Thad's editor more than delivered on his prior promise by hand-delivering himself the initial imprint of Thad's new book. "Kath," said Thad, too frail by then to examine the volume on his own, "you look it over and check to see that it's all OK." After she assured him that it was, Thad asked her to take it, sign it for him, and give it not, for instance, to their seminary's library, but to Dr. MacManus in gratitude for keeping him alive—regardless of the physician's interest in reading "small 'b' baptist" theology.

Thad hung on, semi-conscious, for a week or so. One night, Kath curled up next to him in bed, quietly singing hymns to comfort him until she fell asleep around eleven. When she re-awoke at 4:00 AM, Thad lay beside her dead.

Kath called me that afternoon, a Monday, to tell me of Thad's death. At one point, she tried to console me by saying that "from a 'God's-eye' point of view, God gave Thad long enough and not one day longer, because if the advance copy of his book had come just twenty-four hours later, he would never have had the clarity to appreciate its arrival." But her words, however well-intended, did nothing to bring me solace. They were unable to overcome my hurt, born of my own helplessness. For all my hospice background, for all my training in theology, most of it from Thad himself, I couldn't help this man—teacher, mentor, friend, and father-figure rolled-in-one—relieve his suffering, raise his spirits, or, so far as I could see, remain true to the great story he professed when his own life story neared its end.

Worse yet, I could find no end, no closure, in the story between Thad and me. In our final conversation, four or five days before Thad's death, he ended the phone call with no mention of his illness or his dying, but exactly as he always did: "Well, Michael, it's time for my martini. Lovely speaking with you. I love you, and so does God." In view of all that had occurred, or rather, of all that had *not* occurred, his words rang worse than hollow, as some cliché to cut me off and out. Consequently, when he died, and for a long while later, I could hardly stand the gouge made somewhere deep within me when I remembered all that he had done for me, and all that had been left undone. Ultimately, Thad's disease did more than take its toll upon his heart: it tore the heart out of my relationship with him.

Only nine years after Thad had died did I chance upon a sermon he had given that put some of the heart back in it. Thad had spoken in that sermon of friendship and the ways it might go wrong. One kind of blunder, he noted, grew out of trusting others too little and hence of living within oneself too much. He remarked parenthetically—but tellingly—about that type of fatal friendship flaw: "and I think this is my own." Reading that little line in passing clarified so much for me about *his* passing, about Thad's inability to let me in, not to mention all the others—Kath, their seminary's staff and students, and maybe even God himself.

Thad's sermon, though, had noted another way in which friendship could go awry, underscoring the sort of misstep that I, not he, had made. It lay at the other end of friendship's spectrum, namely, trusting people overmuch, thus entailing, as Thad put it, "the possibility of disappointment or betrayal." And whom had I too readily befriended? I had cozied up too quickly to my own ego, setting too much stock in my ability to make it easier for Thad to meet his death. In the process, I had imagined a scenario more enchanting than any children's fairy tale, where such magical thinking properly belongs. But adults need entirely different stories, cautionary tales that warn us not to think that we can rightly imagine another's death, let alone our own, regardless of whatever greater story we might hope to re-enact as ours draw to a close.

Thus, a story closes this book's narratives of spirits raised and spirits crushed as they were summoned to answer the knocking coming from death's door. The varied accounts of the end of life retold in this book contrast starkly to any and every story that could conclude: "And they all died happily ever after." In that respect, the narratives told here also challenge all the fables of death and dying that purport to furnish some overarching "meaning of human life." The most that these or any such narratives can yield are the multiple meanings of the irreplaceable lives of those who lived them—and of all those others who, having loved them, lamented them once they died. Hence, in the end, this book has offered only stories, inviting its readers to locate themselves within their midst, to rummage through their contents, and to find, perhaps, something that better illuminates a previously faint twist or turn in their own life's storyline.

In the last analysis, we *are* our stories. Our life stories have threads interwoven with those of others, the whole warp and weft forming the fabric of memory, bringing us by turns suffering and succor, despair and consolation. Following some thread of memory, we can trace, if possible, the journey back from the grief of spirits dashed to the hope of spirits healed. Through truthful storytelling, memory may become more a blessing than a curse. So let this, the book's final line, serve as an epitaph for Thad and for all the others whose stories it has told, not inscribed on still and stationary tombstones, but echoed in their survivors' still-beating hearts: "May their memory be a blessing."